THE
**REAL**
TRUTH

# HORMONE
## REPLACEMENT

D0817078

# DR SANDRA CABOT

# HORMONE
# REPLACEMENT

## HOW TO **BALANCE** YOUR
## HORMONES NATURALLY

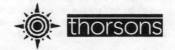

Thorsons
An Imprint of HarperCollins*Publishers*
77–85 Fulham Palace Road
Hammersmith, London W6 8JB

The website address is www.thorsonselement.com

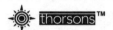

and *Thorsons* are trademarks of
HarperCollins*Publishers* Ltd

This Thorsons edition published 2004

I

First published 2002 by WHAS Pty Ltd.
P. O. Box 689
Camden NSW, 2570 Australia
Phone 00 612 4655 8855
Email – cabot@ozemail.com.au
www.weightcontroldoctor.com
www.liverdoctor.com

Cartoons by Karen Barboutis

A catalogue record for this book
is available from the British Library

ISBN 0 00 717897 2

Printed and bound in Great Britain by
Clays Ltd, St Ives plc

## Disclaimer

The suggestions, ideas and treatments described in this book must not replace the care and direct supervision of a trained healthcare professional. All problems and concerns regarding your health require medical supervision by a medical doctor. If you have any pre-existing medical disorders, you must consult your own doctor before following the suggestions in this book. If you are taking any prescribed medications, you should check with your own doctor before using the recommendations in this book.

## Dedication

This book is dedicated to all the wonderful women on the planet who deserve to enjoy their golden years in a civilized way.

## About the Author

Dr Sandra Cabot MBBS, DRCOG, is a medical doctor who has extensive clinical experience; she treats patients with hormonal imbalances, chronic diseases and weight problems.

Dr Cabot works with other medical doctors and her team of naturopaths; her practices are situated in Camden and Edgecliff, Sydney, New South Wales, Australia.

Dr Cabot began studying nutritional medicine while she was a medical student, and has been a pioneer in the area of holistic healing. She graduated in medicine with honours from the University of Adelaide, South Australia in 1975. During the 1980s she worked as a volunteer in the largest missionary Christian hospital in India, tending to the poor indigenous women.

Dr Cabot pilots herself to many cities and country towns in Australia where she is invited to speak at seminars and exhibitions.

Her free magazine, called *Ask Dr Sandra Cabot*, can be read on-line at www.weightcontroldoctor.com

# Contents

# Introduction:

## My Perspective on Arriving at the Menopause

When I was a young woman, I considered women of 40 to be old, and I related best to women of my own age group. I enjoyed delivering babies and dealing with gynaecological problems, and considered helping women to go through the menopause to be less of a challenge.

I never looked forward to getting older, and I associated the process of ageing with a loss of power and vitality. As a child I related to Peter Pan – he could fly anywhere and had magic powers. Peter Pan never got old, and neither would I!

When I turned 50, I found that my concepts of ageing were wrong. The day of my 50th birthday I woke up and said to myself, 'Wow! I feel so powerful and energized.' I had so much knowledge to give and share, and I felt inspired to go out into the world and be myself. I felt as though the creative force that keeps me alive and breathing – whether you call it God or the divine force – had entered my being and given me a new sense of direction. I was grateful for this and felt it to be a special gift. This experience happened within me, and was not dependent upon my life circumstances.

A woman of 50 has lived life and has understood so much

that a younger woman has yet to know. Perhaps the milestone of 50 is a sacred rite or passage that needs to be celebrated. By this age we have become women of substance, no longer frightened to show their stuff to the world. Sure, we may have flagging hormones, a few wrinkles on our face, a few spare tyres around our abdomen and a few bones that ache, but wow we have a mind that has become a treasure-house of knowledge and understanding. Yes, we are truly fortunate to be able to live as long as 50, as not all of our sisters get to live this long. I consider that every year I live beyond 50 will be a bonus.

Yes, it is good to be wise and happy when we get to menopause; we deserve this – it is not hard to achieve, as this experience lies within us all – it is a gift and is our divine right.

Now I have arrived at 50, I am complete and fulfilled, proud of my achievements, and I hope to be a humble servant of the greater power that sustains us all. I have come to understand that –

My health is my greatest asset.

I can be happy in myself, irrespective of my relationships.

I can live my life as an expression of myself, and not justify it to others.

I can find love and fulfilment in sharing and helping others.

All the love that I need is found within me, and I do not need to rely on another person to make me happy.

I can have a fulfilling and interesting relationship with my own mind and I do not have to be bored.

I can continue to learn and grow and become a better person.

I do not have to worry, and I am taken care of by something much greater than my own concerns.

There are many philosophies and ideologies, but the soul can only be quenched by love.

I will always be beautiful, although my body will age.

I will always be young in the eyes of our creator, and I can always experience the excitement and adventure of a child.

I value my friends and team of helpers who help me achieve my goals.

I can always believe in my dreams, as only this will make them happen.

Although I need to listen to others, I can trust my own intuition.

I have a unique experience of life that is so special, and so do you – as women we need to stand together and help all our sisters achieve their true potential. It's called woman power and it's great! As they say, 'I don't suffer with hot flushes, I have power surges!'

When we share the truth, we do not have to be academic or intellectual; the truth is the truth – it is honest, makes sense, and is beautifully simple.

Welcome to the truth about HRT and the experience of the menopause!

### It Is Time for a Totally New Approach.

I believe it is time for a totally new and truthful perspective on the menopause. Currently women are confused and are uncertain about what they can or should do about their flagging hormones as they become older. I have helped literally thousands of women go through the menopause over the last 25 years, and I have witnessed many different types of Hormone Replacement Therapy (HRT) come and go. I have been through my own menopause, and you could say I have been through the menopause thousands of times, along with my patients, while trying to help them!

I have used many types of HRT with great success, and I have found that HRT can have a dramatically beneficial result in many women. Different forms of HRT can alleviate the horror of postnatal depression, overcome premenstrual mood disorders, and rejuvenate the sex life of older women. Indeed, I have found that 'hormones make the world go round!' Many of my patients wish to continue with HRT in some form, and come to see me to find out how they can continue to use hormones in a safe, natural way. Many of them are very unhappy about the prospect of completely giving up any form of HRT.

One of the reasons why women are so confused is that there is now so much conflicting information about the pros and cons of different types of HRT; indeed, many women feel that they have too much information to sort through. There are books that tell us that we should avoid ALL types of hormones and rely exclusively upon herbal treatments. There are other books that tell us that all women need ONLY ONE hormone, called progesterone, and that all the other hormones available are unimportant, dangerous or will create imbalances.

None of these theories is strictly correct, because every woman is a unique individual and needs her own tailor-made program to help her through the hormonal upheaval of the menopause and ageing. Some women will find that natural progesterone by itself is totally inadequate; other women will find that herbal formulas alone do not have an adequate effect.

When it comes to hormones, we must always rely on science and safe proven medical practices; however, there is also the art of prescribing HRT, which takes years for a health professional to perfect. All the body's hormones need to be correctly balanced and fine-tuned like the instruments in an orchestra, to enhance the emotional, physical and sexual quality of our lives.

## Some Thoughts at the Menopause

*I have some lines in my face from fifty years of life.*
*They tell me of years in the sun, of sorrows and joys.*
*They tell me of time.*
*They tell me I have lived and that I am still alive.*
*They can't be erased. They can be softened...*
*Do I long for the smooth-skinned, freckle-faced kid I*
  *once was?*
*No. I long for the same thing today that I longed for*
  *then: to be the best I am able to be.*

Taken from Kaylan Pickford, *Always a Woman*
(NY: Bantam Books, 1982)

# Chapter 1

# The History of HRT

Over the years there have been many different studies and clinical trials examining HRT. Some have shown that HRT protects against cardiovascular disease, while others have shown that it increases the incidence of blood clots. Some studies have shown that long-term oestrogen, by itself, increases the risk of breast and uterine cancer, and we now know that combined oestrogen and progestin tablets given for over three years also increase the risk of breast cancer.

## Major HRT Studies: A Summary

1975 – *The New England Journal of Medicine* published the results of two major studies that showed that oestrogen given alone (without progestogens) increased the risk of uterine (endometrial) cancer.

1985 – The US Nurse's Health Study involving 120,000 women found that oestrogen replacement in post-menopausal women reduced the risk of heart disease.

1995 – The US Nurse's Health Study found that oestrogen increased the risk of breast cancer.

1997 – The Collaborative Group on Hormonal Factors in Breast

Cancer found that women on HRT have a three times higher risk of blood clots.

2000 – The National Cancer Institute study found a 40 per cent increase in the risk of breast cancer in women on combined HRT.

2002 – The US Women's Health Initiative (WHI) Study showed that combined oral HRT increased the risk of blood clots, stroke, cardiovascular disease and breast cancer.

In the 1970s we found that oestrogen given alone increased the risk of uterine cancer, so we then added synthetic progestogens to the oestrogen, to stop this danger. However, in avoiding HRT-induced uterine cancer, we then induced even more dangers – namely an increased risk of breast cancer, cardiovascular disease and blood clots. In other words, by trying to prevent one type of cancer, we have introduced a range of different, unexpected problems. The results of the WHI Study show definitively that when synthetic HRT interferes with the balance of the body's natural hormones, we can expect adverse effects in a significant number of women.

## Oral Combined HRT – No Longer the Gold Standard

Oral combined HRT generally consists of tablets containing natural or equine oestrogens, combined with a synthetic progestogen.

The vast majority of the long-term studies of HRT have been done using **hormone tablets**, most of them using equine-derived oestrogens and synthetic progestogens. These studies have *not* examined the long-term risks of natural hormones that are absorbed through the skin, such as gels, creams and patches. Absorption of hormones through the skin is called transdermal absorption, as opposed to oral absorption.

Hormones applied to the skin do not pass through the liver immediately after absorption. There is a huge difference in the metabolic effects of oral hormones compared to hormones that are absorbed through the skin (transdermally).

One of the major reasons that large long-term studies on natural HRT absorbed through the skin have not been done by drug companies is that it is not possible to patent a truly natural hormone. Thus there is no financial incentive for drug companies to do these very expensive studies, as they would never recoup their costs.

Personally I have never felt comfortable prescribing hormone tablets for the long-term treatment of menopausal symptoms. This is because hormone tablets must be broken down by the liver immediately after their absorption from the gut, and thus will exert metabolic changes in the liver. These metabolic changes can increase the production of proteins, including clotting factor proteins by the liver, and this is why HRT given orally will increase the risk of blood clots.

I have also found that oral HRT will cause weight-gain in many women, and that is because it increases the workload of the liver. The healthy liver is the major fat-burning organ in the body; if you increase its workload, there will be less metabolic energy left within the liver cells to burn fat.

Oral combined HRT can increase the incidence of migraines, high blood pressure, high cholesterol, fluid retention and liver and gall bladder problems, once again because of its adverse effect upon liver function.

## How It All Started

Many women are now feeling confused, and no doubt somewhat abandoned, as they learn of new controversies about the hormone tablets they take, which drug companies once promised could protect their bones and hearts from the ravages of time.

Well, let's face it, hormone replacement therapy is nothing

new, and has always been controversial, and either in or out of fashion.

Way back in 1889, Professor Charles Edouard Brown-Sequard announced to the French Academy of Sciences that he had injected himself with testicle juice extracted from the pulverized testicles of guinea pigs. He proudly stated that this testicle juice produced a miraculous rejuvenation in his body! At the time of injecting himself he was 72 years old, and his state of physical exhaustion had led him to experiment with a hormonal treatment. He said that, 'Before I gave myself these injections, I could not work for more than half an hour in the laboratory without having to sit down; even when I was sitting down I felt exhausted after three hours of work. By the third day after starting these injections, all that was changed, and I had recovered my former vigour. I can now without effort or even thinking about it, run up and down the stairs – as I used to do, up to my 60th birthday. After the first two injections, my forearm showed an increase of 6 or 7 kilograms over its previous strength.'

Professor Brown-Sequard was talking about the powerful rejuvenating effect of the hormone testosterone, which was present in abundant amounts in the guinea pigs' testicles. He also obtained excellent results after injecting ovary juice into women. The Medical Record of 20 June 1889 acknowledged that Brown-Sequard's discovery was brilliant, if incomplete. Although he was controversial, in many ways he advanced the speciality of hormones, known as endocrinology, and he was a great researcher.

Progesterone was isolated and collected from the ovaries of pigs, and from human placentas, in the early 1930s. In 1938 natural progesterone was first synthesized from the plant hormone diosgenin, by an American biochemist named Russell Marker.

In the 1940s natural forms of HRT were developed mainly by Schering Pharmaceuticals in Germany, and injections containing natural oestrogen, progesterone and testosterone became popular.

Oestrogen therapy first became famous in 1966, when American doctor Dr Robert Wilson, released his best-selling book *Feminine Forever*, which promoted oestrogen as the elixir of youth. To Dr Wilson, his discovery that oestrogen was able to rejuvenate women's lives was just as momentous as the replacement of insulin in people with diabetes, who could no longer make insulin themselves. In *The Journal of the American Geriatric Society* in 1972, Dr Wilson wrote, 'Breasts and genital organs will not shrivel, and women will be much more pleasant to live with, and will not become dull and unattractive.' I do not think that Dr Wilson's comments would be popular with modern-day women – they are decidedly sexist and ageist!

Professor Brown-Sequard and Dr Wilson were correct – hormones are powerful rejuvenators with anti-ageing effects, and many people have had their lives dramatically improved by the use of natural HRT.

## Changing Attitudes

Compared to 100 years ago, women now have a much longer life span, and go through the menopause at a relatively young age. This begs the question – 'Is it really natural to load up every postmenopausal woman's body with high doses of synthetic hormones for the last 20 to 30 years of her life, just to prevent chronic diseases that may never happen?'

I think to do so is an over-reaction to a normal phase of a woman's life. You could say this approach is not natural nor physiological, and yet during the past 20 years we have come to see this practice as acceptable and even desirable. I think this idea originated in the mid-1980s when the 'medicalization of the menopause' was first promoted. This concept generated fear that women must do something drastic to overcome the 'disease of the menopause'. In 1985, a special supplement in *The Medical Journal of Australia* stated that, 'The post-menopausal climacteric should be regarded as a sex-linked, female dominant, endocrine deficiency **disease**, with specific symptoms and signs, which should be investigated and managed in a very careful and considered fashion, for the remainder of the woman's life.' This concept was promoted to the medical profession, so that doctors started to see the menopause as a disease state, for which they should prescribe therapy. Thus the idea of the menopause as a disease to be feared was passed on to women by their doctors and the media. Women's attitude towards their own menopause started to change, so that they no longer saw it as a natural phase of their lives. This imposed attitude was a barrier to women seeking to get in touch with their own feelings and reactions towards the menopause. They started to see hot flushes as a symptom of disease, and the term 'the change' became synonymous with the beginning of a downward spiral. This atmosphere of fear made many women feel that without dependence upon long-term medicines, their own actions could not have a significant impact on their future health. Thus the mid-1980s was a time of disempowerment for older women. They were mistakenly led to believe that the prevention of the diseases of ageing – namely heart disease and osteoporosis – could **only** be successfully controlled by HRT, and not with self-help measures such as a healthy diet and lifestyle.

All women were put into the same 'herd mentality', and the concept of treating all menopausal women the same was created; in other words, 'one-brand one-dose of HRT' was thought to fit all women. The concept of 'super-market-brand-name-HRT' became entrenched, and the last 30 years of a woman's life was now a lucrative commodity.

I was never impressed with this concept, as I could see that many of my patients were unsuited to oral synthetic hormones. My suspicions about oral HRT were confirmed when, as a young doctor in the 1970s, I visited the retirement haven of Miami Beach in the US. During the 1970s, the Premarin brand of oestrogen was the fifth-biggest-selling prescription drug in the US. In Miami Beach I observed thousands of older women enjoying their golden years who had been, or were taking, the fashionable HRT. However, these women did not look healthy – their skins were wrinkled and their postures stooped, and they lacked vitality. Unfortunately the elixir of synthetic hormones could not undo the damage from years of inactivity, smoking and consuming refined processed foods. Interestingly, during the 1980s when I worked in a missionary hospital in northern India, the older women looked much stronger and more youthful than those in Miami Beach, despite a life of hard work, no HRT and nutritional restrictions.

During the 1990s, HRT continued to increase in popularity, and in the year 2000, 46 million prescriptions were written for Premarin (equine oestrogens), making it the second most frequently prescribed medication in the United States, accounting for more than $1 billion in sales, and 22.3 million prescriptions were written for Prempro (Premarin plus Provera). The US Food and Drug Administration approved this type of HRT for the relief of menopausal symptoms and the prevention of osteoporosis, and long-term use of HRT became fashionable to prevent a range of chronic diseases, especially heart disease.

## Women Want Choices

All of the millions of women out there who have been happily taking oral combined HRT now find themselves in a dilemma. Many feel they have been misled or abandoned, however the current situation is a reflection of the fact that research takes many years to give us long-term results. Well, we do not want to be research guinea pigs! Now is the time for women to stick together and explore the safest and most natural options. Yes, it is a time where common sense and instincts should prevail, and luckily you do not have to be a rocket scientist to see that there is a world of difference between the different types of HRT now available. Indeed, you do not even have to be a doctor!

This book will take away the fear and confusion surrounding HRT and the menopause, and bring you right up to date. There is no doubt that **certain types of HRT** can help to slow down the ageing process and improve the quality of your physical, mental and sexual life.

There is no need to give up all hope; some forms of HRT may be able to help you, with minimal risk involved. In other words, you don't have to throw the baby out with the bath water!

Very few things in life are risk free or come with a 100 per cent guarantee, so let's get real! We all take a calculated risk every time we drive a car, play sports or, indeed, leave the house. You can even get robbed while you are still at home, and you can never indemnify your life completely. Most of us want to live life to the full and feel challenged, stimulated and sensual, so we take calculated risks every day.

If we can relieve the unpleasant symptoms of the menopause and ageing with effective treatments that do not expose us to unacceptable risks, then we have achieved the best possible compromise. By understanding the ways that natural HRT can be given without upsetting the body's natural equilibrium, we increase our choices of strategies that will safely improve the quality of our lives.

Some women will not need any HRT, and will need instead a good diet and healthy lifestyle. Other women will find that the menopause and ageing process produce undesirable and/or painful changes in their body and mind, which can only be relieved with some form of natural HRT.

Thankfully, the menopause is no longer 'the change of life'

that is to be feared. I often reflect upon just how difficult it must have been for women who lived in the early 1900s to cope with these unpleasant symptoms. They must have been very strong women indeed, but strength alone cannot get you through severe hot flushes, insomnia, a desolate sex life, fibromyalgia or a severe emotional imbalance. These women had no choices – no HRT, no anti-depressant medications and probably very little understanding from society, the medical profession or their families.

Today, women have vastly different expectations of life, and do not want to suffer unnecessarily with unpleasant symptoms. They do not want osteoporosis, rapid ageing or an unsatisfying sex life.

Since the 1940s, HRT has gone through many trends, fashions and different types of packaging. We now have so many ways of putting hormones into your body that it is quite incredible! This ranges from hormone tablets, implants, injections, pessaries, vaginal rings, patches, creams, gels, sprays and lozenges (troches). Among all these possible ways of taking HRT, it is now possible to find a safe tailor-made programme of HRT to suit every woman who wants to take HRT.

Thankfully, the woman of today has access to natural HRT, modern-day drugs and nutritional medicines that can alleviate the symptoms that were once considered the hallmark of the beginning of ageing. Yes, we are truly fortunate to be living in this day and age!

## The Modern-day Controversy about Hormones

Before the results of the Women's Health Initiative (WHI) Study were published in August 2002, millions of women in the UK, US and Australia were using some type of HRT.

The use of non-hormonal alternatives for the menopause has also increased. It is true that drug companies have a vested interest in the lucrative baby-boomer generation of women, and it is true that women also have a big interest in a type of HRT that will promise them a better quality of life. However, the baby-boomer generation of women is well educated and discerning, and wants to know the real facts.

Thus, the results of the WHI Study on the effects of combined oral HRT on 16,000-plus women was very timely, and have proven to be a defining moment in medical history that could be considered a bombshell for many researchers in the field of HRT.

The Study uncovered some alarming findings that obviously worry doctors and consumers of HRT. The data and safety monitoring board recommended stopping this trial prematurely because women receiving the active hormones had an increased risk of invasive breast cancer, and an overall measure suggested that the HRT was causing more harm than good. The decision to abandon the trial occurred after an average follow-up period of 5.2 years, although the trial was originally planned to continue for 8.5 years. There were other outcomes that suggested danger, such as an increased risk of coronary heart disease and pulmonary embolism.

Overall, the results of the WHI Study confirmed the growing body of evidence that combination oestrogen/progestin tablets can increase the risk of breast cancer with increasing duration of use, and increase the risk of stroke and blood clots during five years of use. The increased risk of coronary heart disease was largely found during the first year of HRT use. Overall, this American study found that women on combined oestrogen and progestin tablets had a 26 per cent increased relative risk of developing breast cancer, a 29 per cent increase in heart disease, and were 41 per cent more likely to have a stroke. Most of these problems began appearing within the first one to two years of HRT use, but the increased breast cancer risk did not begin until three years of use.

Positive effects of the combined HRT regime were a reduction in the risk of bowel cancer and bone fractures.

In terms of absolute risk, the above figures can be translated into the following statistics – if 10,000 women take combination oral HRT for one year, eight more will get invasive breast cancer, seven more will have heart attacks, eight more will have strokes, and eight more will have blood clots, compared to a similar group of women not taking the hormones. On the plus side, there will be six fewer cases of bowel cancer and five fewer hip fractures.

You can see from these absolute risks of harm, when we look at 10,000 women taking HRT for one year, the risk to an individual woman is not great. However, if we count all the adverse health events that happened over the 5.2 years of the WHI Study, the excess number of adverse events in the women using the HRT was 1 in 100 women. This is a small risk, but shows that risks from combined oral HRT add up over time.

Although the WHI Study was set up originally to demonstrate the ability of HRT to prevent common diseases of ageing, the Study found that the opposite effect appeared to be happening. Given these results, the authors of the Study are recommending that doctors stop prescribing combined oral HRT therapy for long-term use.

Since the results of the WHI Study have caused such a furore, many people are asking questions that will take time to answer definitively – it is possible that future studies will find that the benefits outweigh the risks, perhaps thorugh the use of different combinations or formulations of more natural hormones. For example, studies are needed to determine the long-term benefits of transdermal natural hormones provided as patches or creams. I am confident that these will be shown to be safer than oral combined synthetic HRT, but only time will tell.

Professor Graham Colditz from Harvard Medical School was refreshingly candid about the results of the WHI Study: he said they are a major wake-up call to both consumers and health authorities. Since the WHI Study was abandoned, Professor Colditz and many other health experts around the world **no longer recommend the use of long-term combined oral HRT to prevent disease.** However, the use of combined oral HRT is still considered as generally safe when used for **short-term** treatment to **relieve** menopausal symptoms. My attitude to this is – Why would you use oral synthetic hormones when you have natural hormones that can be given in a more physiological way to relieve the symptoms of menopause?

The results of the WHI Study were based upon using 0.625 mg of Premarin (conjugated equine oestrogen) plus 2.5 mg of Provera (medroxyprogesterone acetate). Other types of oral hormone combinations may have different results. However, three studies using other oral combinations of HRT have all found an increased risk of breast cancer. An Oxford University Study in the mid-90s showed that oral HRT increased the risk of deep vein thrombosis. A long-term study of nurses found a link with breast cancer in 1995, but until now, the risk of combined oral HRT has generally been kept rather low key in mainstream medicine. Well, we have known for years that oral oestrogens such as Premarin, if taken for more than five years, will increase the risk of breast cancer by around 30 per cent. So why has the outcome of the WHI Study created such a bombshell?

It could be partly because the experts cannot seem to agree on the significance of the findings of the WHI Study –

Dr Deborah Grady, Director of the Mount Zion Women's Health Clinical Research Center at UCLA (University of California in Los Angeles), believes that the results of the WHI Study provide compelling evidence that doctors find a way to get women off oestrogen.

Dr Maura Quinlan, an HRT specialist at the University of Chicago Hospitals, states 'We have to stop using HRT for healthy women.'

Dr David Dammery, a GP and chairman of the Victorian College of General Practitioners in Australia, is very much against HRT for long-term prevention.

Other well-known professors world-wide believe that the design of the WHI Study was flawed, and that its results are not representative of the true value of HRT in healthy menopausal women. They criticize the sample of women chosen in the WHI Study as being unsuitable candidates for the use of HRT in the prevention of cardiovascular disease. They cite the problem that the sample of women chosen was too old and unhealthy to be used in a primary-prevention trial of the benefits of HRT.

Indeed, 66 per cent of the women in the WHI Study were 60 years or older. One-third of women in the study sample were obese, 36 per cent were being treated for high blood pressure, 12.5 per cent were being treated for high cholesterol, and 50 per cent were ex-smokers. Thus they were not representative of healthy women who had just arrived at menopause. According to these experts, the results of the WHI Study are not meaningful for healthy post-menopausal women. They also point out that there was no increased death rate among the women in the WHI Study who took HRT, compared to those who did not.

## What Are the Real Issues?

As a doctor who sees thousands of peri-menopausal women, I believe that it is the quality of life now, and in the immediate future, that is most important to women. This is what women grapple with every day, and it greatly affects the enjoyment of their lives.

Just because **certain types of hormones** have been found to be unacceptably dangerous for long-term use, does not take away the need for, and interest in, hormone replacement therapy. Women are not so much interested in how they will feel in 20 or 30 years' time, but rather want to be able to enjoy the still relatively young years, at least in today's terms, that exist between the ages of 45 to 65. Also, today's woman is smart and well educated and wants to know ALL her options. She knows that osteoporosis and heart disease have much more to do with diet and lifestyle than with hormones. The reality is this – if you have a poor diet, are overweight, smoke heavily or do not exercise, then all the HRT in the world is no guarantee that you will be saved from diabetes, fractures and heart attacks. Yes, a magic HRT pill to protect us from ageing and disease would be great – I would take it! However, we are all too smart to be duped by the drug companies.

The issues of the moment for peri-menopausal women are:

How do I feel and look today?
How does my mind function?
Do I have energy and vitality?
Do I feel sexual, sensual and feminine?
Can I have a good sexual relationship with my partner?
How can I remain healthy for the next 20 years?

To help women achieve their goals and satisfy the above expectations, doctors have to think laterally, practise holistic medicine and have empathy with every individual woman. If this is not their area of interest, they can always refer to a doctor who is interested in this sub-speciality of medicine. Clinical trials are based upon large numbers of subjects, statistics and a generalized deduction and recommendation. However, many individual women do not really relate to this academic world – it can be frightening and confusing for women trying to relate to the academic ivory tower.

First we must be honest with women – they deserve it! They depend upon doctors and we want to keep their trust.
Women would like to know that:

- Very few pharmacological treatments in medicine are perfect – most are a compromise between relief and possible side-effects. We need to weigh up all the pros and cons. If we do take HRT it will have a protective effect upon our bones and usually improve our sex life, however if we use a potent oral form of HRT for more than several years, it may increase our risk of blood clots, strokes and breast cancer.
- There is a great difference between individual women – some women need HRT to enjoy their lives, while others feel well and function efficiently without HRT. We should not frighten all women off HRT – some types of HRT remain a viable and safe option for many women.
- Nutritional medicine can work, especially for the prevention of long-term degenerative diseases; however it cannot simulate the effect of real hormones in the way we feel. For example, homoeopathic hormones do not work at all, and herbal hormones will not achieve the exact same effect of real hormones.
- There is a huge difference in the effect induced in the body by different types of hormones. For example, hormones taken orally, as in the WHI Study, are absorbed from the gut and pass straight to the liver. The liver breaks the hormones down (metabolizes them) and only a certain amount gets past the liver into the general circulation; thus we must use higher doses of more potent hormones to gain a clinical result. This increases the workload of the liver, and induces the liver enzymes to make more clotting factors; thus we become more at risk of blood clots and heart disease. Also, because the progesterone that is commonly used in oral HRT is synthetic, it takes longer to be broken down by the liver, and may accumulate in the body, causing more side-effects. I have never thought that it was physiological (natural) to give hormones by mouth for this reason, unless we require oral contraception. It is much more physiological to give hormones in a way that bypasses the liver. To achieve this, we must

administer hormones through the skin (which is called transdermal administration), via implants, sprays, vaginal creams or rings, or injections. Transdermal administration can be achieved by using hormone creams, gels or patches. Some doctors use lozenges (troches) that are designed to be placed between the upper gum and the cheek, so that the hormones they contain are absorbed directly into the blood vessels under the lining of the cheek. This way we are meant to avoid swallowing the hormones and thus absorbing them from the gut and then through the liver. Some women tell me that it is difficult to avoid swallowing some of the lozenge, especially since they come in several hundred delicious flavours!

I personally feel more comfortable prescribing transdermally-absorbed hormones via the creams and/or patches, especially for long-term use or for women with risk factors for HRT. The beauty of the creams is that they can be tailor-made for the individual woman, to contain the combination of natural hormones that she needs as determined by her blood tests, medical examination and history.

- Although there are some very favourable clinical trials evaluating the use of hormone creams for various hormonal problems, there are no very long-term studies available on their safety for use as HRT for the post-menopause.
- The use of any form of HRT is the choice of the patient, and it must be based upon informed consent. Women need to know that we cannot give them 100 per cent guarantees of safety, and that, generally speaking, it is wise to find the lowest dose of HRT that will relieve unpleasant symptoms and improve well-being. This can be compared to taking the oral contraceptive pill – women know about the risks, as they are printed on the packet. However, millions of women choose to take the Pill, because its advantages often outweigh the disadvantages in the individual woman.

Communication is the key – doctors need to treat women as intelligent human beings. Women need to take some responsibility in helping their doctor to decide if they will use HRT. They can only do this if they know and understand all their options. Luckily you do not have to be a rocket scientist to work out the advantages of different types of HRT. Common sense and realistic expectations should be explored. It is always possible to prescribe HRT for a short period (less than a one year), choosing a transdermal application just to see if it really makes a difference. Then you can weigh up the absolute risks, if any, of long-term use before deciding whether to continue.

Just because yet another hormone controversy has raised its head does not mean that all women will stop wanting to take HRT. Today's menopausal woman has a much longer life span, and totally different expectations of life, than women who lived 100 years ago. She does not want to –

- age rapidly
- stop being sexually alive
- embrace old age mentally and physically at the tender age of 50.

There is no doubt that hormones can help us feel and look younger and keep us sexually young. Just imagine if men ran out of their sex hormones at the tender age of 50 – well, there would be a hormone shop in every suburb!

Yes, 'hormones make the world go round' and, controversial or not, they are not going to become strictly taboo!

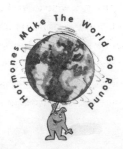

# Chapter 2

# The Menopause

The average age of the start of the menopause is 51; however, some women will go through the menopause many years earlier than this. Fertility starts to decline after the age of 35, due to the gradual reduction in the number of healthy follicles (eggs) in the ovaries. The incidence of hormonal imbalances is more common after the age of 35, simply because the ovarian follicles are ageing.

You are more likely to experience Premenstrual Syndrome (PMS) during the years from age 35 up to the menopause. This is because, after ovulation, the ovaries may not always produce adequate amounts of the female hormones called oestrogen and progesterone.

*During the peri-menopause it is more common for progesterone production to be inadequate, which can result in symptoms of relative oestrogen excess such as:*
- heavy and/or painful menstrual bleeding
- growth of fibroids and uterine polyps
- growth of endometriosis
- irregular menstrual cycles
- premenstrual depression and mood disorders

- premenstrual headaches
- fluid retention
- abdominal bloating
- breast tenderness and lumpiness
- hair loss

## The Peri-menopause

This phase of a woman's life is defined as the several years before and after the menopause. Hormonal imbalances are common during the peri-menopausal years.

The menopause is said to have occurred when menstrual bleeding has been absent for 12 consecutive months. Because the age of the menopause varies considerably, the time of onset of the peri-menopause also varies. The majority of women will go through the menopause between the ages of 45 and 55.

The years following the menopause are called the post-menopause. During the post-menopause, the production of sex hormones from the ovaries continues to decline, and may eventually become non-existent.

## What Causes the Menopause?

The human female is the only creature known to live much longer than her sex glands and reproductive capacity. We could ask 'Why us and not men?' or 'Did Mother Nature have a design fault?'

These questions are valid, however the fact remains that our ovaries simply run out of follicles (eggs). It is the follicles that produce the vast majority of the female sex hormones, and thus we are no longer able to produce these hormones in adequate quantities. The age at which the supply of ovarian follicles becomes exhausted varies between women; this is why we see such a large variation in the age at which the menopause occurs.

## IS THERE A TEST FOR THE MENOPAUSE?

The menopausal ovary being devoid of follicles is unable to manufacture significant amounts of the female sex hormones. If a blood test is done to measure the levels of oestrogen and progesterone, they will be found to be at very low levels. In menopausal and post-menopausal women, blood oestrogen levels (which are measured in the form of oestradiol) are generally less than 160pmol/L. The term pmol/L means picomoles per litre, and is a standard laboratory measurement.

### Typical Results of the Hormone Levels in Menopausal and Post-menopausal Women

| HORMONE | BLOOD LEVEL |
|---|---|
| FSH | greater than 30U/L |
| Oestradiol | less than 160pmol/L |
| Progesterone | less than 3nmol/L |

Oestradiol is the most potent form of oestrogen produced by the ovary. Other types of oestrogen produced by the ovary and the fat tissue are weaker, and consist of oestrone and oestriol.

The function of the ovaries is under the control of the pituitary gland, which is situated at the base of the brain and acts as a master-controller for the most of the hormonal glands in the body. The glands which produce hormones are known as endocrine glands, and the medical speciality of hormones is called endocrinology.

The pituitary gland is very sensitive to the hormonal output of the ovaries, and it begins to react when the ovaries fail to pump oestrogen and progesterone into the bloodstream. Indeed, the pituitary gland is not at all 'happy' with the failure of the menopausal woman's ovaries. The pituitary gland quickly responds by pumping out large amounts of a hormonal messenger called Follicle Stimulating Hormone (FSH).

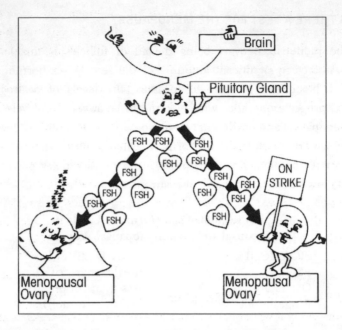

FSH travels from the pituitary gland, via the bloodstream, to the failing ovaries to try to stimulate them back into action.

Alas, this does not work; the ovaries have 'closed up shop' forever, and despite the hormonal pleas and wooing from the pituitary gland the ovaries remain inactive. Meanwhile, the pituitary gland cannot comprehend that the ovaries are unable to respond to its advances, and in a futile attempt to reawaken them it continues to pump ever-increasing amounts of FSH into the bloodstream. This achieves nothing as far as the ovaries are concerned, but it does provide a useful diagnostic test for your doctor to determine if you are menopausal. Typically the blood FSH levels are quite high if you are menopausal, and will be greater than 30 U/L, and may reach up to 300 U/L. In other words, you will have **continually elevated levels of FSH**, and this is the **most accurate test for the menopause.** Obviously all women who are wondering if they are menopausal will want to know what their FSH level is, because if they are truly menopausal they no longer have to worry about contraception. They will also know if it is the failure of their ovaries that could be responsible for any unpleasant symptoms that they may be suffering with.

If you are on the oral contraceptive pill, you will need to stop taking it for several months before having a blood test; otherwise your blood tests for the menopause will be inaccurate. The oral contraceptive pill makes the results of blood tests for hormone levels totally meaningless. Women on the Pill will **always** show very low levels of both FSH and their own naturally-produced hormones, because the Pill suppresses the production of hormones from the pituitary gland and the ovaries. I am often amazed that women are sent for testing of their hormonal levels while they are still taking the Pill!

## Symptoms of the Menopause

Some women will not experience any menopausal symptoms and may get a shock to discover that their blood tests show menopausal levels of hormones!

Other women may experience unpleasant symptoms, ranging from mild to severe, such as:

- Hot flushes
- Aches and pains – sometimes called fibromyalgia
- Vaginal dryness and discomfort
- Vaginal shrinkage
- Painful sexual intercourse
- Bladder problems such as urgency and incontinence
- Loss of sex drive
- Shrinkage of the breasts
- Mood changes, which may be severe enough to result in a clinical depression
- Low self esteem

- Anxiety and panic attacks
- Memory problems
- Poor concentration
- Dry and ageing skin
- Hair loss
- Sleep disorders

These symptoms may come on gradually during the peri-menopausal years, or may come on quite suddenly. Understandably they can be very distressing, especially if you do not understand what is causing them.

To assess your level of oestrogen and progesterone deficiency, blood tests and/or salivary tests are very accurate.

You can also take a minute to fill in the questionnaire below, which is known as 'Your Oestrogen Level Score Chart'.

If your total score for all of these symptoms is 15 or more, then it is likely that you are suffering from a deficiency of oestrogen.

If your score is 30, your body is probably crying out for oestrogen. This can be confirmed or refuted by a simple blood test to check your levels of oestrogen and follicle-stimulating hormone (FSH).

It is an interesting exercise to score your symptoms of oestrogen deficiency before and after starting HRT. Computing your score every three to four months provides a useful self-check to see whether your hormone replacement therapy is adequate. However, you should not decide to alter your dosage based on the results of this questionnaire without first consulting your doctor.

## OESTROGEN LEVEL SCORE CHART

| Symptom | Your Score |
|---|---|
| Depression and/or mood changes | _____ |
| Anxiety and/or irritability | _____ |
| Feelings of being unloved or unwanted | _____ |
| Poor memory or concentration | _____ |
| Poor sleeping patterns | _____ |
| Fatigue | _____ |
| Backache | _____ |
| Joint pains, arthritis | _____ |
| Muscle pains | _____ |
| Increase in facial hair | _____ |
| Dry skin and/or sudden development of wrinkles | _____ |
| Crawling, itching and/or burning sensations in the skin | _____ |
| Reduction in the sexual desire | _____ |
| Frequency of or burning sensation with urination | _____ |
| Discomfort during sexual intercourse | _____ |
| Vaginal dryness | _____ |
| Hot flushes and/or excessive sweating | _____ |
| Lightheadedness or dizziness | _____ |
| Headaches | _____ |
| **TOTAL SCORE** | _____ |

The symptoms that are characteristic of oestrogen deficiency can be grouped together in the chart above, and scored according to the following scale:

Absent = 0      Mild = 1      Moderate = 2      Severe = 3

## How Long Does the Menopause Last?

The word 'menopause' means the cessation of menstrual bleeding – that is, the last menstrual period. When this occurs your ovaries no longer contain any viable eggs (follicles), and so they can no longer produce significant amounts of sex hormones. So no more eggs means no more hormones, and technically we could say that once the menopause has arrived, it is here to stay.

However, the menopause is not a disease – it is merely a state of relative sex hormone deficiency; we do not want women to think that now they are menopausal, they have incurred a permanent disease that requires long-term medical intervention.

During the early 1980s I worked in a missionary hospital in India, which I found a fascinating anthropological and spiritual experience. Luckily I spoke some Hindi and had a solid training in Obstetrics and Gynaecology, as we were presented with all sorts of female emergencies that are no longer common in Western countries. I was in my early 30s at the time, and although I knew how to deliver babies and treat gynaecological problems, I was still very naive about the ways of the world and about cultural differences. I was quite surprised to find that Indian women saw the menopause as a completely different experience to the majority of my patients in Australia. Indian women welcomed the menopause and saw it as a liberating time in their lives; they no longer had to worry about unwanted pregnancy, continual anaemia from menstrual bleeding and childbirth, and the load of a big family. However, their liberation was not due to the loss of fertility alone, it was also because they were now free to be themselves. I found that many of the older Indian women, even up to their late 70s, were still sexually active, notwithstanding their lack of HRT. They were pleased to be able to have their vaginal and bladder repairs done, not just to overcome urinary incontinence but also to feel good about themselves as women, and also so they could have a better sex life. So this experience taught me a lot – the way we see the menopause has a lot to do with the expectations that have been brainwashed into our subconscious minds. The menopause is just a new phase of life, and really we are lucky to be able to live long enough to experience it!

Some women will have very few menopausal symptoms, and so the time that the menopause lasts becomes quite insignificant. In those women who continue to experience symptoms of hormonal deficiency right up into their late years, we can use either nutritional medicine or a combination of natural HRT and nutritional medicine to relieve their symptoms completely. So although the menopause is a permanent stage of your life, any unpleasant symptoms do *not* have to be permanent.

HRT can be taken for a short period of time, or for many years. We now know that oral forms of oestrogen and/or progestogens are not safe to take for more than several years, due to the increased risk of breast cancer and blood clots. They can be taken for one to two years, if you prefer to take oral forms of HRT.

If HRT is to be used for many years to relieve unpleasant symptoms in older women (over 55), then I personally believe that the natural forms of oestrogen, progesterone and testosterone, administered in the form of creams, patches or low-dose lozenges (troches) are a very safe alternative. As a woman ages, she will generally need smaller doses of HRT, and the amount of hormones in the creams can be easily adjusted accordingly. In many cases it is only necessary to use the creams in the vaginal area, making the amount of hormones absorbed into the bloodstream much lower.

### What Are the Myths Surrounding the Menopause?

Many women are reluctant to consider HRT anymore, because of sensational media coverage, or books they may have read. However, many of these things are nothing more than hormonal myths. Below we look at some of these common misconceptions, as well as the true facts about HRT.

| MYTH | TRUTH |
|---|---|
| If I start on HRT, I will never be able to come off it. | Not true, HRT is not addictive. |
| Homoeopathic hormones such as DHEA and melatonin will relieve my symptoms as well as real hormones do. | Homoeopathic hormones do not work like real hormones, as they are present in infinitesimal doses. |
| Herbal preparations are converted into real hormones in my body. | There is no proof that herbal hormones can be converted in the body into real hormones. |
| Natural HRT is the same as herbal hormones (phytoestrogens). | Not true, natural hormones are human hormones and some require a doctor's prescription. |
| HRT should always be taken for the shortest possible time. | If we use small doses of natural hormones that are administered via the skin or vulva, they can be used for long periods of time. |
| HRT never causes weight gain. | If potent hormones are given orally, they may cause weight gain in some women. |
| Menopause is a short phase of my life. | Menopause is a permanent state of relative sex hormone deficiency. |

| MYTH | TRUTH |
|---|---|
| Blood tests are not an accurate way to tell if I have become menopausal. | It is necessary to check the FSH levels. |
| I will not need any HRT until after my periods have finished completely. | Some women need natural progesterone to help balance their hormones, well before the menopause arrives. |
| Once I lose my sex drive, there is nothing I can do about it. | Wrong, natural HRT, used in the correct way, can make you sexually young again. |
| All HRT will definitely increase my risk of breast cancer. | Small doses of natural hormones in the form of creams or patches have not been shown to increase the risk of cancer. Natural progesterone and oestriol may exert anti-cancer effects. |
| All HRT will definitely increase my risk of blood clots and strokes. | Natural HRT given in a way that bypasses the liver, such as in patches or creams, has not been shown to increase blood clots or strokes. |
| I am too old to take HRT. | Possible benefit from HRT has little to do with your age, but rather your lifestyle, sexual needs and symptoms. |

| MYTH | TRUTH |
| --- | --- |
| If I take HRT, I do not need to take a calcium and mineral supplement. | It is always vital to take a good calcium-mineral tablet, as this will improve bone density and will reduce your risk of osteoporosis. HRT alone is not adequate to protect against osteoporosis. |

## What Tests Should I Have During the Menopause?

- Every peri-menopausal woman should have a Dexa Bone Mineral Density test to determine her risk of osteoporosis. If bone density is abnormally low, the test should be repeated regularly, either annually or biannually.
- She should see her doctor every 12 months for a breast examination and a vaginal and pelvic examination.
- A mammogram and pap smear should be done every two years.
- Blood pressure measurement, weight, urine and cholesterol testing should be done annually.

### A Menopause Examination Checklist

This table provides you with a general checklist of important tests that are often performed at the menopause, together with what the doctor is looking for when doing them. Your doctor will decide if any special tests, such as blood tests or pelvic ultrasound, are needed in your individual case.

| EXAMINATION | WHAT THE DOCTOR LOOKS FOR |
|---|---|

**THE PHYSICAL EXAMINATION**

| | |
|---|---|
| Heart, blood pressure, blood vessels | High or low blood pressure; signs of cardiovascular disease; varicose veins. |
| Weight | Underweight; obesity. |
| Thyroid gland | Enlargement; lumps. Under or overactivity can be confirmed with a blood test for thyroid function. |
| Breasts | Lumps; thickening; skin or nipple changes. |
| Abdomen | Swelling; tenderness. |
| Pelvic examination | Size of pelvic organs; condition of ovaries; signs of cancer, prolapse of uterus or bladder, vaginal atrophy. |

**SPECIAL TESTS**

| | |
|---|---|
| Pap smear | Cancerous or precancerous cells in the cervix. |
| Mammogram | Very early signs of breast cancer. |
| Bone mineral density test (BMD) | Signs of osteoporosis. |
| Blood count; blood tests for oestrogen, follicle-stimulating hormone (FSH), blood sugar, liver function, cholesterol level | Blood oestrogen level; signs of metabolic disorders. |

| | |
|---|---|
| Urinalysis | Signs of infection, kidney disease. |
| Pelvic ultrasound | Signs of disease of the uterus and/or ovaries. Pelvic ultrasound is useful for women in whom pelvic examination is difficult, uncomfortable, or inconclusive. |

# Chapter 3

# Hormonal Imbalances

## How Hormones Work

### Oestrogen Dominance

You may have heard of the term 'oestrogen dominance' and wondered what it is. Some doctors use this term, which describes the effect of a relative excess of oestrogen in the body compared to progesterone.

This can be caused by over-production of oestrogen in the body, or a deficiency of progesterone. During the pre-menopausal years, due to ageing of the ovaries and infrequent ovulation, it is common for women to produce adequate oestrogen but not enough progesterone. Oestrogen dominance can also be caused by the oestrogenic effects in the body of xenoestrogens, which are chemicals derived from petro-chemicals and oestrogens used in the mass production of some meats.

### SYMPTOMS OF OESTROGEN DOMINANCE

- weight gain around the buttocks, hips and thighs
- fluid retention
- abdominal bloating

- lumpy, tender breasts
- heavy and/or painful periods
- irregular or infrequent periods
- endometriosis
- fibroids
- endometrial hyperplasia and an increased risk of uterine cancer

The condition of oestrogen dominance can be confirmed by finding pre-menopausal levels of FSH (less than 20) combined with low levels of progesterone and normal-to-high levels of oestrogen in a blood test. This can also be confirmed with saliva tests.

## WHAT CAN YOU DO ABOUT OESTROGEN DOMINANCE?

- Use natural progesterone in doses of 25 to 100 mg daily for two weeks of every month, or for the last two weeks of the menstrual cycle.
- Increase fibre in the diet, as this lowers oestrogen levels.
- Improve the liver function, as the liver breaks down the excess oestrogen into the weak water-soluble oestrogen called oestriol, so that it can be excreted in the body via the urine.
- Reduce your exposure to xenoestrogens – see page 51.
- Eat only organic eggs and organic chicken.
- Increase your consumption of foods containing phyto-estrogens, such as beans, whole flaxseeds, alfalfa, peas, lentils and vegetables.

### Summary of What You Can Do about Hormonal Imbalances

- **Balance your diet** – Eat more plant-based foods, especially beans of all varieties, alfalfa sprouts, raw nuts and ground whole flaxseed.

- **Use herbal formulas** containing phytoestrogens from mixtures of Black Cohosh, Hops, Liquorice root, Red Clover, Wild Yam, Kelp and Horsetail. These can be found available combined with vitamins and minerals in one capsule.
- **Maintain a healthy weight** through a balanced diet and regular exercise programme.
- **Use more feminine oral contraceptives** such as Marvelon, Femoden, Minulet and Trioden.
- **Use natural hormones** instead of synthetic hormones – such as progesterone cream or progesterone lozenges for premenstrual syndrome or peri-menopausal hormonal imbalances. Use Hormone Replacement Therapy (HRT) that is more natural and does not overwork the liver. Creams containing mixtures of natural hormones, and hormone patches, do not overwork the liver.
- **Consider adrenal gland exhaustion**, a common cause of chronic fatigue, which can be helped with antioxidants such as vitamins C and E, flaxseed oil and the minerals selenium and magnesium. In stubborn cases of adrenal gland exhaustion, the natural adrenal gland hormones such as DHEA and pregnenolone, can produce excellent results.
- **Reduce your exposure to alcohol**, as women who drink more than two glasses of alcohol a day may be increasing their risk of breast cancer. Avoid smoking, as this reduces the production of hormones from the ovaries and adrenal glands.
- **Avoid over-exposure to toxic chemicals**, which are foreign substances called xenobiotics. Xenobiotics are petrochemical compounds found in plastics, solvents, pesticides, herbicides, emollients and adhesives. Over the last 100 years they have become prevalent in household items, garden chemicals, insecticide sprays, plastic pipes and containers, various creams and shampoos, food and water supplies. These xenobiotics are toxic to humans and animals, and result in disruption of the

hormonal system and an increased risk of cancer. In the excellent book titled *Our Stolen Future* by Theo Colborn, documentation is given about the effects of xenobiotic exposure in the early life of wildlife populations; it explains how these chemicals produce a large variety of congenital abnormalities. Petrochemicals are fat-soluble and accumulate in the fatty parts of the body, such as the endocrine glands, where they cause hormonal imbalances and dysfunction. The liver is the only organ in the body that can break down these petrochemical xenobiotics, so it is imperative to support your liver function in this toxic day and age. See www.liverdoctor.com.

## How Are Hormones Made in Our Glands?

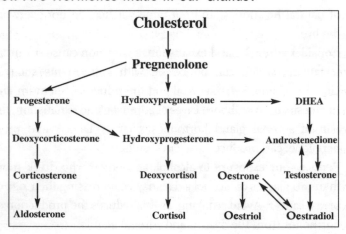

All of our steroid hormones, including the sex hormones, are made in the body from cholesterol. Cholesterol is a sterol that is found in foods of animal origin and is vital for health. If you did not have any cholesterol in your body, you would not make any steroid hormones, including the sexy ones! Thus it does not surprise me when patients on cholesterol-lowering medication, which stops the liver from making cholesterol, complain of a big reduction in their sex drive.

The liver and some parts of the intestine manufacture cholesterol, and if you do not eat any cholesterol-containing foods, your liver will make extra cholesterol to compensate for this.

As seen in the diagram above, cholesterol is first converted into the hormone called pregnenolone. Pregnenolone can be considered a 'mother hormone', as it can be converted into many other types of steroid hormones. For example, pregnenolone can be converted directly into the female hormone progesterone, or it can follow another biochemical pathway and be converted into cortisol. Pregnenolone can also take another pathway and be converted into DHEA, which can then be converted into all the different types of male and female sex hormones. Pregnenolone is a vitally important hormone, as it is the hormone from which ALL the other steroid hormones, including the sex hormones, are made. It could be asked, then, 'Why don't we give pregnenolone alone, so that the body can convert it into all the other steroid sex hormones as we need them?' Unfortunately, as we age the enzymes that are required to convert pregnenolone into the other hormones like DHEA and progesterone also decrease, and become less efficient. Thus it is necessary to replace the specific hormones that are found to be deficient.

The production of steroid hormones from cholesterol occurs in the ovaries, testicles, adrenal glands and, to a much lesser extent, in the fat tissue of the body. Lower-level body fat produces predominantly oestrogen in the form of oestrone, whereas upper-level body fat produces predominantly male hormones. This is why women with excess weight in the upper part of their body, around the trunk and abdomen, often have quite high levels of male hormones, even years after the menopause.

After the menopause occurs, the ovaries no longer produce adequate amounts of the sex hormones. If the adrenal glands are healthy, they will continue to produce some of these steroid hormones, especially pregnenolone and DHEA. This is why women who have healthy adrenal glands will have less severe hormonal symptoms during the menopause. In patients with adrenal gland exhaustion, the hormones DHEA and pregnenolone can be administered, often with excellent results.

The following table gives you, at a glance, the symptoms of imbalances in the hormones oestrogen, testosterone and progesterone.

| HORMONE | SYMPTOMS OF EXCESS | SYMPTOMS OF DEFICIENCY |
|---------|--------------------|------------------------|
| OESTROGEN | Fluid retention | Hot flushes |
| | Breast pain and swelling | Night sweats and insomnia |
| | Heavy menstrual bleeding | Vaginal dryness and discomfort |
| | Painful menstrual bleeding | Vaginal shrinkage |
| | Weight gain in the hips and thighs | Vaginal infections |
| | Headaches and migraines | Painful sexual intercourse |
| | Aching legs and aggravation of varicose veins | Loss of libido |
| | Growth of fibroids and endometrial hyperplasia | Inability to orgasm |
| | Growth of endometriosis | Urinary frequency and/or incontinence |
| | Increased risk of cancer of the breast and uterus | Dry and wrinkled skin |
| | | Depression and anxiety |
| | | Memory loss |
| | | Lack of menstruation |
| | | Bone loss and loss of teeth |
| | | Muscular aches and pains (fibromyalgia) |

| HORMONE | SYMPTOMS OF EXCESS | SYMPTOMS OF DEFICIENCY |
|---|---|---|
| TESTOSTERONE | Hair loss from the scalp<br>Excess facial and body hair<br>Pimples or acne<br>Greasy skin and hair<br>Excess sex drive<br>Weight gain, especially in the trunk and abdomen<br>Elevation of cholesterol<br>Aggressive moods | Shrinkage of muscles<br>Weakness of muscles<br>Loss of sex drive<br>Inability to orgasm<br>Depression and anxiety<br>Loss of confidence and panic attacks<br>Muscular aches and pains (fibromyalgia)<br>Bone loss<br>Fatigue |
| PROGESTERONE | Depression<br>Sleepiness and feeling too relaxed<br>Fluid retention<br>Abdominal bloating<br>Constipation | Breast pain and lumpiness<br>Hair loss<br>Heavy menstrual bleeding<br>Growth of fibroids<br>Growth of endometriosis<br>Endometrial hyperplasia<br>Increased risk of cancer of the uterus and breast<br>Premenstrual mood disorder, depression and anxiety |

| HORMONE | SYMPTOMS OF EXCESS | SYMPTOMS OF DEFICIENCY |
|---|---|---|
| PROGESTERONE (cont.) | | Premenstrual fatigue<br>Menstrual irregularity<br>Absent menstruation<br>Exacerbation of pre-<br>   menstrual asthma<br>    and epilepsy<br>Exacerbation of<br>   multiple sclerosis |

## What Can You Do If You Have Too Many Male Hormones?

If you have excessive amounts of male hormones (androgens) in your body, you may notice several things:

- excess facial and body hair (hirsutism)
- loss of scalp hair, especially in the male pattern of balding
- greasy skin and/or pimples
- difficulty losing weight, especially from the trunk and abdomen

The hormonal profile of a woman going through the menopause, and after the menopause, can vary greatly, and this is why blood and/or saliva tests are so useful, to pinpoint your individual hormonal profile. Some women will have elevated levels of androgens even many years after they go through the menopause. These androgens are produced from the fat in the upper body and abdomen, and also from the adrenal glands. Obviously women with elevated levels of their own natural androgens do not need to receive any testosterone therapy, and usually find that synthetic progestogens make their hormonal imbalance worse. This is because synthetic progestogens may exert a mild androgenic effect. Natural progesterone does **not** have any androgenic effects, and should be used in women with excess androgens who need HRT.

The blood test that is most accurate to detect raised levels of the androgens is called the Free Androgen Index (FAI). This measures the amount of active androgens, which are unbound to proteins and are thus free to exert their effect in the body. If your FAI level is elevated, it is definite that you have excessive male hormone activity in your body. If you do not have any troubling symptoms and are not overweight, then this is not really a problem and you do not need to worry about it; however very high levels of male hormones should always be investigated by a specialist endocrinologist.

I have found that many women with an elevated FAI have normal blood levels of total testosterone, and thus just by measuring total testosterone levels alone you cannot get an accurate diagnosis of androgen excess. You must ask your doctor to order a Free Androgen Index (FAI) test if you want an accurate diagnosis.

*Strategies for Women with Symptoms of Excess Androgens*
- Weight loss from the upper body and abdomen will reduce the production of androgens from the fat tissue.
- Creams or troches containing natural oestrogens and progesterone can reduce the dominance of the androgens, thus making the hormonal profile more feminine.
- If the androgen excess is severe and is producing marked symptoms, the anti-male hormone called Cyproterone acetate can be prescribed. Cyproterone acetate comes in the form of 50-mg tablets. The dose of cyproterone can vary from ¼ of a tablet (12.5 mg) to one tablet (50 mg) daily. Cyproterone also acts as a progestogen, and as such can be given along with oestrogen to balance the effect of oestrogen on the uterus. If cyproterone is

given every day, then there will not be any bleeding; if you desire to have a regular period, then the cyproterone can be given cyclically, for 18 days of every calendar month, along with your oestrogen. You must avoid pregnancy while taking cyproterone acetate. Generally speaking cyproterone is well tolerated, especially if the dose is tailor-made to match the patient's blood tests and the severity of her symptoms. If the correct dose is used, then cyproterone will reduce the action of the male hormones so that we achieve a big improvement in all the symptoms of excessive androgens. Interestingly, we find that in women whose obesity is associated with excess androgen levels, the use of cyproterone will aid weight loss. This is because high levels of androgens will aggravate the high insulin levels found in Syndrome X. Syndrome X is a chemical imbalance that makes your body store fat and prevents your body from burning fat. If too much cyproterone is given, the level of the body's androgens will be reduced too much and the patient may complain of fatigue, depression and loss of libido. As with all forms of hormone therapy, it is vital to tailor-make the correct dose for each patient, and over time the dose may need further adjustment.

# Chapter 4

# Testing for Hormonal Imbalances

## When Can Hormone Tests Be Useful?

- To determine if you are menopausal. Blood tests are better for this initial test, to check your FSH levels and baseline levels of total sex hormones.

- During the pre-menopausal years, if you have heavy and/or painful menstrual bleeding, fibroids or irregular menstrual cycles, as this could indicate a progesterone deficiency. The best time to measure progesterone levels is seven days before your menstrual bleeding is due, although if your cycle has become irregular and/or infrequent, it can be difficult to pinpoint this exact time. Salivary and blood tests should be done to check progesterone levels.

- If you are on hormone replacement therapy, to indicate if your response to treatment is adequate. These tests can be blood and/or saliva tests. The blood tests are done every three to six months; the saliva tests can be done more often. The tests are more necessary if you are on HRT and you still feel that your hormones are out of balance. For women on higher-dose forms of HRT, such as implants or injections, blood tests can be helpful to check that you are not receiving an excessive dosage. We do not want to produce very high blood levels of hormones that are above the normal ranges, so blood and saliva tests can check for over-dosing as well as under-dosing. If you are on HRT and feel well, you may not need any hormone tests at all.

## Useful Blood Tests and their Normal Ranges During the Menopause

| HORMONE | COMMENTS | NORMAL RANGE DURING THE MENOPAUSE |
|---|---|---|
| Free testosterone | Measures the free component of testos-terone, which is the active hormone. | Blood: 0.5 to 6pmol/L |
| DHEA – Sulphate | Measures the reserve amounts of DHEA. | Blood: 200 to 2700ng/ml or 0.5 to 7.3umol/L |
| Oestradiol | Blood tests measure the total circulating amount of the most powerful oestrogen, called oestradiol. | Blood: less than 150–200pmol/L in menopausal women not receiving any HRT. |
| Progesterone | Blood tests measure the total circulating amount of Progesterone, and not the free active component. | Blood: less than 3nmol/L in menopausal women not receiving any HRT. |

| Cortisol | Blood tests measure the total circulating amount of cortisol. Cortisol is made in the adrenal glands. Normally the levels of Cortisol are higher in the early hours of the day. | Morning: Blood: 220–720nmol/L Evening: Blood: 110–390nmol/L |
|---|---|---|
| Thyroid Stimulating Hormone TSH | TSH is a pituitary hormone which becomes elevated if the thyroid gland is underactive. | Blood: 0.3 to 5.0 mIU/L |
| Free T 4 | This blood test measures the circulating amount of the free T4 hormone. The free component is the active hormone. | Blood: 9.0 to 24.0 pmol/L |
| Free T 3 | This blood test measures the circulating amount of the free T3 hormone. The free component is the active hormone. | Blood: 2.2 to 5.4 pmol/L |
| FSH | FSH is a pituitary hormone which | Blood: 30 to 280 U/L in menopausal |

| | | |
|---|---|---|
| FSH cont. | becomes elevated once the menopause arrives. | women not on any HRT |
| Free Androgen Index (FAI) | This is a very useful blood test. The FAI measures the total amount of all the free androgens circulating in the bloodstream. This test accurately measures the activity of the male hormones in the body. The FAI may be elevated even if the levels of testosterone are normal, and provides a more accurate assessment of excess androgen activity in the body than measuring testosterone does. | Blood – 1 to 8 % |
| Testosterone | Measures the total amount of testosterone in the blood. | Blood – less than 1.0 to 4.5nmol/L |
| Sex Hormone Binding Globulin (SHBG) | Measures the amount of  globulin protein in the blood that binds the sex hormones. | Blood – 30 to 90nmol/L |

According to some experts, the dose of oestrogen required in HRT should be sufficient to improve cellular activity but not excessive enough as to create an abnormal response from the liver. The conventional oestrogen doses commonly used in the past were considered to be effective if they produced blood levels of oestradiol within the range of 150 to 1000umol/mL. Blood levels towards the higher limit of this range can easily be achieved with oestradiol implants and injections, or tablets of Premarin 0.625 mg and Progynova 2 mg daily, and the stronger oestrogen patches.

However, for most women it is not necessary to produce blood levels of oestradiol over 300 to obtain relief of symptoms. We do not want to have blood oestradiol levels continually as high as 1000 umol/mL, as this may increase the risk of oestrogen-dependent cancers; a high dose of synthetic progestogen would be needed to balance these high oestrogen levels. These high blood levels of oestrogen often result in 'oestrogen dominance' with symptoms of oestrogen excess such as fluid retention, nausea, migraines, breast swelling and tenderness, and abdominal bloating. When we use the lower doses of natural oestrogen in the form of creams or lower-dose patches, much lower doses of natural progesterone are adequate to balance the oestrogen.

Furthermore, by using oestrogen creams or patches we are able to bypass the liver so that higher levels of the free active oestrogen are available to the cells. In this way we are able to avoid producing high levels of total oestrogen in the blood.

## Is Testing Hormone Levels in the Saliva Accurate?

Salivary hormone levels are tested by conventional and complementary healthcare practitioners to assist with hormonal balancing in their patients.

Saliva test and blood test results do not always match up, especially as far as progesterone is concerned. This is because progesterone binds to the red blood cells in the bloodstream.

Before the blood levels of progesterone are measured, the laboratory spins off and discards the red blood cells so that **only** levels of progesterone remaining in the serum are measured. This will give a falsely low reading in the blood tests for progesterone levels, so that women using progesterone creams, and their doctors, get the wrong impression that the progesterone is not being absorbed into the body. If this is so, then a more accurate response to the progesterone cream can be obtained with a saliva test.

Salivary hormone levels measure accurately the **free or available** amount of sex hormones in the body.

Conversely, the sex hormones found in the blood serum are largely bound to protein and are not readily available to the body's cells. Indeed, 90 to 99 per cent of the sex hormones in the blood are bound to carrier proteins (such as cortisol-binding globulin, sex-hormone-binding globulin and albumin), and are unavailable to act on the body's cells and perform their functions. **Blood levels of oestradiol, progesterone and testosterone** are mostly a measure of protein-bound hormone, and **are useful to determine how much total hormone is present in the body.** Blood levels of hormones are preferable when we want to measure the total amount of hormones circulating in the bloodstream.

Some medical experts believe that blood tests for sex hormones are irrelevant, because they measure the protein-bound (non-available) hormone **plus** the free non-protein-bound (available) hormone, and not the free hormone by itself. I disagree with this, because I think it is useful and important to know the total amounts of hormones in the body, as this reflects the amount of hormone produced or administered. However, it is true that the free component of the hormones readily filters into the saliva. The measurement of the free, and thus the active hormones is easily measured with saliva tests. Saliva is an excellent medium to measure steroidal hormones, as they are not bound by carrier proteins and are therefore free and bio-available.

# Summary of the Benefits of Testing the Salivary Hormones

- The fraction of hormone measured in the saliva is the free and unbound, bio-available hormone (i.e. it is not bound to a carrier protein).
- Saliva testing is non-invasive, economical and can be done in the privacy of your own home. Saliva samples are returned to the laboratory for analysis.
- Saliva collection does not require special handling.
- Baseline hormone levels can be assessed, and natural hormone replacement therapy can be easily monitored and adjusted.
- Multiple saliva samples can be taken in a single day or over a number of weeks (and frozen) to evaluate hormone levels.
- Salivary hormone tests currently available can test the levels of the hormones oestradiol, progesterone, testosterone, DHEA-S, cortisol and melatonin.
- Salivary hormone testing is available for men and women (see www.betterhealth.ltd.uk/tests).

Salivary hormone testing is used to guide supplementation dosages and to determine if natural hormone replacement therapy is being absorbed.

For example, maintaining appropriate levels of both oestradiol and progesterone is important, as an excess of oestradiol can lead to 'oestrogen dominance' and cause symptoms such as breast tenderness, heavy and/or painful periods and weight gain in the hips and thighs. In such cases, saliva testing shows us that it is necessary to reduce the dose of oestrogen and/or increase the dose of natural progesterone.

# Reference Ranges of Hormones Measured in Saliva

| Hormone | Female Follicular | Female Luteal | Postmenopausal | Male |
|---|---|---|---|---|
| **Oestradiol** | 2–10 pmol/L | 6–14 pmol/L | 2–8 pmol/L | <10 pmol/L |
| **Progesterone** | 50–200 pmol/L | 140–520 pmol/L | 50–200 pmol/L | <125 pmol/L |

| Hormone | Female | Male |
|---|---|---|
| **Testosterone** | 25–190 pmol/L | 100–400 pmol/L |
| **DHEA-S** | 2.5–25 nmol/L | 5.0–30 nmol/L |

| Hormone | Time of day | Levels |
|---|---|---|
| Cortisol | 0700–0800 | 5.3–61.8 nmol/L |
| Cortisol | 1900–2000 | 1.2–12.3 nmol/L |
| Melatonin | 2200–0700 | 10–40 pg/mL |
| Melatonin | 0700–1300 | <3.0 pg/mL |

*Note:*

The follicular phase is the first half of the menstrual cycle before ovulation occurs in a pre-menopausal woman.

The luteal phase is the second half of the menstrual cycle after ovulation occurs in a pre-menopausal woman.

After menopause ovulation ceases, and so these phases of the menstrual cycle become non-existent. During the post-menopause, the natural hormone levels remain at consistently low levels unless HRT is given.

Scientific references for salivary hormone testing are available on the website www.arlaus.com.au, which can help patients to understand their saliva test results more easily.

## Interpretation of the Salivary Hormone Tests

| Hormone Tested | To Assess |
|---|---|
| **Progesterone, Oestradiol Testosterone (men and women)** | The function of the ovaries and testicles. The effectiveness of Hormone Replacement Therapy. |
| **DHEA & Testosterone (men & women)** | To check the function of the adrenal glands and testicles. To evaluate the effectiveness of Hormone Replacement Therapy. |
| **Cortisol & DHEA** | The function of the adrenal glands looking for underactive states (such as adrenal gland exhaustion and Addison's disease) or over-active states such as Cushing's disease. Also to check the adrenal gland's response to stress. |
| **Melatonin** | Looking for problems with the body's biorhythms and the cause of some types of insomnia and depression, such as seasonal affective disorder. |

# Chapter 5

# The Ins and Outs of Natural HRT

## What Is the Difference between Natural and Synthetic Hormones?

This is a very common question, and is a point of confusion for many women.

### NATURAL HORMONES

Natural hormones are chemically identical to the hormones produced by your own glands, which means that your body cannot tell the difference between your own hormones and a natural hormone prescribed by your doctor. These natural hormones are called **bio-identical hormones**.

Natural hormones are made in the laboratory from a plant hormone called diosgenin, which is extracted from yams and soybeans. By making slight physical changes to the diosgenin's molecular structure, we are able to turn diosgenin into natural human hormones such as oestrogen, progesterone, etc.

If you take a look at the diagram below, you will see that diosgenin has a similar chemical structure to natural oestradiol and progesterone, so that only relatively minor changes need to be made to diosgenin to turn it into these human hormones.

We are able to synthesize the following natural **bio-identical hormones** from plant hormones:

- progesterone
- the three types of oestrogens – oestriol, oestrone, and oestradiol
- testosterone
- DHEA
- pregnenolone
- androstenedione.

These natural hormones can be administered in the form of creams, gels, lozenges, tablets, capsules, patches, implants, injections and pessaries.

The comparison of the chemical structure of an Isoflavone and the sex hormones Oestradiol and Progesterone

Many women think that natural hormones are found only in herbs, plants and foods, and that any hormone that is synthesized in a laboratory must be synthetic. However, all natural prescription hormones, including those in creams and lozenges, are synthesized in a laboratory. In the laboratory a plant hormone can be turned into either a natural or a synthetic hormone; it is the final molecular structure of the hormone that is important.

The characteristic of a hormone that makes it qualify as a natural hormone is not its origin, but is its final molecular structure. Provided a hormone has the exact molecular structure, as a hormone produced naturally in the human body it can be classed as natural.

## SYNTHETIC HORMONES

These have a different chemical structure to your body's own hormones, and are more difficult for the liver to break down (metabolize). This makes synthetic hormones much stronger than natural hormones, and also more likely to cause side-effects. Sometimes this increased potency can be desirable when we need to use strong synthetic hormones to overcome severe endometriosis or to reduce dangerously heavy menstrual bleeding. The hormones used in the oral contraceptive pill need to be synthetic because natural hormones are not strong enough to prevent ovulation from occurring. However, where possible it is safer and better accepted by the patient to use natural hormones when treating problems such as premenstrual syndrome, post-natal depression, post-tubal ligation problems and the menopause.

### What Are the Latest Ways of Taking Hormones?

Many of the letters and emails I receive are from women who complain that conventional oral HRT does not really work as they had hoped it would. In other words, conventional medicine often misses out when it comes to prescribing 'the right stuff'. For some women, brand name HRT does not really work as anticipated, because it is **not** tailor-made for your individual needs. Conversely, with tailor-made HRT we take into account:

- your body weight and body type
- your emotional and sexual needs
- your personal history
- your medical problems and risk factors
- your unique metabolic and hormonal characteristics
- the results of your blood tests and/or saliva tests
- your family history.

Not all women are suited to the standard doses of the HRT brands of Premarin 0.625 mg and Provera 2.5 mg daily, which is how HRT has most commonly been prescribed in the past. This type of standard treatment has been prescribed because of the results of clinical trials and studies that have used the same type and dose of HRT for every woman, irrespective of her body type, weight, age, blood tests and metabolism. Thus you can understand why the results obtained from these trials, such as the WHI Study, are limited and can be misleading. There is an urgent need for more ongoing studies which look at the long-term use of natural hormones prescribed in the form of creams, troches and patches. In these trials the type of HRT should be individualized for every woman, and that is why these trials are more difficult to do. Furthermore, drug companies cannot patent the natural hormones, so there is less financial incentive for these companies to spend millions to undertake these trials. Most of the brands of progesterone used in conventional, standard HRT contain synthetic progesterone, which is called a progestogen. These progestogens do not act like natural progesterone in the body, however; they attach themselves to the progesterone receptors and stimulate or block them. They can cause mood disorders, weight gain and coronary artery spasm, and undo the good effects of oestrogen on the cardiovascular system. In some cases progestogens can also elevate the bad LDL cholesterol and lower the good HDL cholesterol.

The cross-species oestrogen called Premarin, which comes from pregnant mare's urine, is metabolized into more potent compounds which increase your risk of oestrogen dominance. So why would women want to take molecules that their body was never designed to handle?

The art and science of natural HRT has blossomed in the last five years, and we can now tailor-make combinations of natural hormones to suit every individual woman. Thankfully, the old-fashioned style of 'supermarket HRT', where the menopause was treated with stock-standard doses and brands of hormones, is no longer considered desirable by women.

It is only in the last decade that compounded lozenges (troches) and creams containing natural hormones have become generally available. The beauty of the hormone creams and patches is that smaller doses of the hormones can be used, because these types of hormones bypass the liver. Indeed, taking sex hormones by mouth is generally an inefficient way to take them. This is because the liver and intestines break down the majority of the hormones before the surviving hormones can enter the bloodstream. This loss of hormones is known as the 'first pass loss' phenomena. Furthermore, taking hormones orally increases the liver's production of the binding protein SHBG, which binds and inactivates the hormones; thus we get a greater reduction in the immediate action of the hormones.

Giving hormones through the skin is far more efficient because the hormone is absorbed in its free form directly into the bloodstream. This explains why the amount of oestradiol in the patches is 10 to 20 times less than that given in oestradiol tablets.

Progesterone is highly soluble in the fatty layer underneath the skin, and then passes gradually into the capillaries and then into the bloodstream. This avoids 'first pass loss' in the liver, and thus we need only use approximately one-quarter of the dose in a cream, compared to a capsule, troche or tablet of progesterone. For more accurate dosing, salivary levels of progesterone will need to be monitored.

Oestrogen therapy is sometimes also available in the form of a nasal spray which contains oestradiol hemihydrate. Some women get relief of hot flushes with very small doses of this nasal spray, taken in a dose of one puff in each nostril daily. The spray cannot be used by women with nasal problems such as allergic inflammation of the nose. I personally would prefer the use of oestrogen creams to a nasal spray, because other natural hormones can be added to a cream.

During the first few years after the menopause, prescriptions for HRT often need to be fine-tuned with regular adjustments in the doses of the various hormones. This is because a woman's body, symptoms and sexuality are continually evolving as she ages. The goal of natural HRT is to restore body hormones to levels that relieve symptoms. An integrative balanced or holistic approach, considering the possible need for all three classes of sex hormones (oestrogen, progesterone and androgens) is ideal, even in women who have had a hysterectomy. Currently many women who have had a hysterectomy are offered only oestrogen, without consideration of the need for natural progesterone or androgens. Many different combinations of hormones – including the three types of natural oestrogens, natural progesterone, testosterone and DHEA – can be administered in different ways such as patches, tablets, capsules, injections, creams, implants and lozenges (troches). Because there are so many choices I recommend beginning with a blood and/or saliva test, to evaluate your own hormonal profile before starting any HRT. Ideally treatment should start with low doses of hormones which can be adjusted to find the lowest dose needed to alleviate symptoms. Thankfully, the use of hormone replacement therapy is no longer like 'a bull in a china shop'!

## Natural Oestrogen

There are three types of oestrogen that are produced in the female body:

- Oestrone (E1)
- Oestradiol (E2)
- Oestriol (E3)

The predominant natural oestrogen made by the ovary is oestradiol, which is rapidly broken down into the weaker oestrogen called oestrone. Oestrone is broken down into the much weaker oestriol, which is excreted unchanged in the urine. Oestrone is produced in significant amounts in body fat, which is one reason that bigger women often have a later menopause, have less osteoporosis and do not have such severe symptoms of the menopause. Conversely, women who are underweight with low body fat will often have more severe menopausal symptoms, and require higher doses of HRT.

The most commonly prescribed forms of oestrogen used in HRT are oestradiol and oestrone, which are available in a wide variety of forms. The weakest of all the body's oestrogens is oestriol, which makes it a good choice for women who want to use the lowest possible amounts of oestrogen.

Doctors who prescribe natural hormones may use different combinations of the three types of oestrogens in any one cream or lozenge.

Triest is a mixture of oestrogens often used in creams or troches; as its name suggests, Triest contains three types of natural oestrogen in the following ratios:

- 7% Oestradiol (E2)
- 3% Oestrone (E1)
- 90% Oestriol (E3)

Some pharmacists will use a Triest with a slightly different ratio of the three oestrogens.

Generally speaking, a total daily dose of 2.5 mg of Triest is equivalent to 0.625 mg of Premarin.

The ratio of oestrogens in the Triest is designed to mimic the proportions of the natural oestrogens produced by the ovaries.

Biest is a mixture of oestrogens often used in creams or troches; as its name suggests, Biest contains two types of natural oestrogen, in the following ratios:

- 20% Oestradiol (E2)
- 80% Oestriol (E3)

Biest is more potent than Triest, as it contains more oestradiol, the strongest of all the three types of naturally-occurring oestrogens.

You can see that in the Triest and Biest formulations, the predominant oestrogen is oestriol. The rationale for this is that some research has shown that oestriol exerts an anti-cancer effect. The other two oestrogens, namely oestrone and oestradiol, are added to the oestriol because the oestriol by itself does not appear to maintain bone density. This is the most important reason to combine oestriol, with its protective benefits, with smaller amounts of oestradiol and oestrone. When natural progesterone is added to the oestriol, we also get an augmentation of positive effects upon bone density.

Some women will find that all they need to use is an oestrogen cream in the vagina and on the vulval area. If you have a uterus, you must use some progesterone with this oestrogen cream, either in the form of troches or a progesterone cream.

This is because the use of oestrogen alone, in women who have a uterus, can result in over-stimulation of the uterine lining, leading to endometrial hyperplasia.

One advantage of oestrogen replacement therapy is that it elevates the good cholesterol (HDL) and promotes healthy blood vessel walls; this is why oestrogen replacement has been linked in the past with a reduced risk of cardiovascular disease. However, if oestrogen is given in tablet form it may increase the risk of blood clots. Furthermore, if oral oestrogens are given with synthetic progesterone tablets, there will be an increased risk of cardiovascular disease. This is because the synthetic progesterone (progestogen) reverses the good effect of oestrogen upon the blood fats. According to the well-known Australian cardiologist Dr Ian Hamilton Craig, oestrogens have a number of protective effects against atherosclerosis, and natural progesterone may also protect against coronary heart disease.

Oestrogen reduces the rate of bone loss, although by itself it will not build bone. Progesterone and testosterone are also beneficial for bone density.

Women in their late fifties and sixties will often want to continue with some form of nutritional and/or hormonal support for the post-menopausal years, with the aim of reducing osteoporosis and cardiovascular disease. During these two decades the body produces fewer and fewer sex hormones, and this can cause continuing bone loss, increased cholesterol levels and sexual dysfunction. In these older age groups, lower doses of oestrogen replacement are required, and this is ideally given in the form of patches or creams. If older women are troubled by sexual and/or bladder dysfunction, creams combining small doses of oestrogen, testosterone and progesterone, applied to the vagina and vulva, work extremely well. These types of hormones, combined with pelvic floor exercises, can help to reduce common bladder problems such as cystitis, urinary frequency and incontinence.

## Natural Progesterone

This hormone has been discussed in the Table on page 233. Progesterone has really been in the limelight lately, with several eminent researchers promoting its benefits.

The true pioneer of natural progesterone is the British physician Dr Katarina Dalton. Dr Dalton wrote many books on natural progesterone, including *Once a Month*, and her books remain in print. I first became aware of Dr Dalton's books during the 1970s; to me they were like a bolt of lightning – here at last was a powerful female doctor offering the first real, natural solution for premenstrual mood disorder and post-natal depression.

Dr Dalton treated many thousands of women with natural progesterone, and found that it was effective for:

- premenstrual mood disorder
- premenstrual epilepsy and asthma
- post-natal depression
- many gynaecological problems.

Progesterone is needed to balance the effects of oestrogen. Oestrogen causes the cells lining the uterus to divide and grow, whereas progesterone inhibits this growth. Oestrogen can be described as a fertilizer, progesterone as the lawn mower. Thus progesterone is needed to oppose the stimulatory effects of oestrogen on the uterus.

The mechanisms that progesterone uses to keep oestrogen in check are:

- Progesterone reduces the oestrogen receptors' stimulating effects upon cancer-promoting genes.
- Progesterone promotes the conversion of the stronger oestradiol to the weaker type of oestrogen called oestrone.
- Progesterone reduces the number of oestrogen receptors

on the cells, thus reducing the sensitivity of the cells to oestrogen.

These are all very important balancing actions, and this vital role of progesterone explains why **all** women who are given oestrogen should always be given progesterone (preferably the natural form) as well, even if they have had a hysterectomy. Natural progesterone is also needed for healthy bone tissue, probably because it stimulates the bone-building cells (called osteoblasts).

Progesterone is only produced from the ovaries after ovulation. Disorders of ovulation are common, and many women ovulate only irregularly, infrequently or rarely, especially as they approach the pre-menopausal years. The most common cause of infrequent or absent ovulation in pre-menopausal women is polycystic ovarian syndrome (PCOS). In pre-menopausal women who have ovulation problems, oestrogen is produced from the ovary but there is no progesterone, or only inadequate amounts of progesterone are produced. The amounts of progesterone are insufficient to balance the oestrogen – this causes the situation of unopposed oestrogen. This oestrogen will stimulate the lining of the uterus to grow thicker, and the lack of progesterone means that the lining can become abnormally thick – this is called endometrial hyperplasia. Women with this condition often complain of very heavy menstrual bleeding with large clots.

If this hyperplasia becomes chronic, pre-malignant changes may occur in the cells lining the uterus – this is called atypical hyperplasia. Around 20 per cent of women with atypical hyperplasia will go on to get uterine cancer, if this problem is not treated.

By administering progesterone (natural or synthetic), endometrial hyperplasia can be prevented, or even reversed. Thus progesterone has an anti-cancer effect.

A study published in *The Journal of the Climacteric & Postmenopause Maturitas* (vol. 20, 1995, pages 191–198) provides convincing evidence that natural progesterone can control endometrial hyperplasia. In this study, 78 premenopausal women with endometrial hyperplasia were treated from the 10th to the 25th day of their menstrual cycle with a vaginal cream containing 100 mg of natural micronized progesterone. This progesterone therapy achieved a complete regression (reversal) of the hyperplasia in 90.5 per cent of cases. During treatment there was a significant reduction in the amount, duration and frequency of the menstrual bleeding. Other good news is that minimal side-effects were observed during this trial, which is in contrast to synthetic progestogens, which commonly produce side-effects.

The researchers concluded that vaginal administration of natural progesterone is:

- effective in treating hyperplasia
- safe to use, because it does not exert unfavourable changes on the blood levels of cholesterol.

This is in contrast to synthetic progestogens, which may exert adverse changes upon cholesterol levels.

Thus, natural progesterone administered vaginally should be considered as a serious alternative to synthetic progestogens in clinical practice, especially in women with metabolic disorders such as polycystic ovarian syndrome, Syndrome X, diabetes, hypertension, fatty liver and problems with levels of blood fats.

Progesterone can also be given in a micronized form (ultra-fine consistency), which means that the progesterone particles are much smaller. This is done to improve absorption from the gut. Micronized progesterone is administered in capsules. A dose of 200 mg of micronized progesterone, given for 15 days per month, is considered equivalent to 10 mg of the synthetic progestogen called Provera (see Table on page 237). If the natural progesterone is given in a dose of 100 mg daily for

25 days per month, this is also considered equivalent to 10 mg of Provera.

Micronized progesterone was evaluated in the Post-menopausal Estrogen/Progestin Intervention (PEPI) Trial.

The PEPI Trial showed that 200 mg of natural micronized progesterone, given for 12 days of the month, was sufficient to prevent over-stimulation of the uterus by Premarin.

The micronized progesterone was shown to have a more favourable effect upon blood levels of cholesterol than the synthetic progestogens. Because natural progesterone is more effective in correcting the adverse changes that occur in cholesterol levels after the menopause, it should be safer than synthetic progestogens when it comes to reducing the risk of heart disease. The micronized progesterone was found to be as effective as the synthetic progestogens in opposing the effects of oestrogen on the uterus.

Doctors have been educated to use synthetic progestogens in HRT for menopausal women. However, now that the WHI Study has shown that synthetic progestogens are not desirable for long-term use in HRT, many doctors will be looking towards safer solutions, such as natural progesterone.

Natural progesterone does far more than just replace the use of synthetic progestogens; it has several powerful health-promoting benefits in itself:

- helps to preserve bone density
- exerts a favourable effect upon the nervous system
- exerts an anti-cancer effect against some types of cancer
- reduces some gynaecological problems such as fibroids and endometriosis.

Natural progesterone has very different effects to synthetic progestogens in the body, and is far less likely to produce unpleasant side-effects. For example, synthetic progestogens can increase

the risk of spasm in the coronary arteries, whereas natural progesterone reduces such spasms. Natural progesterone is a smooth muscle relaxant and thus usually helps to reduce menstrual cramps.
Synthetic progestogens are far more likely to produce side-effects
such as weight gain, depression, fluid retention, headaches and
breast tenderness. This is because the synthetic progestogens
increase the workload of the liver, as they must be broken down by
the detoxification-pathways (cytochrome P-450 enzymes) in the liver.

The synthetic progestogens fit into the progesterone receptors (and often some of the androgen receptors) on the cell
membranes. This means that they block these cell receptors
from the action of natural hormones.

## What Is the Difference between Hormone Troches and Creams?

Generally speaking I prescribe creams containing natural hormones before I prescribe troches (lozenges). This is my personal preference; other doctors will use troches more than creams
to administer HRT.

Both the creams and troches can be made up to contain any
combination and varied amounts of natural hormones. In other
words, exactly the same types and same amounts of hormones
can be put into a troche or cream.

Generally speaking the troches are stronger (more potent)
and are more likely to cause breakthrough bleeding than the
creams are, although they can be designed to produce a regular
menstrual bleed if preferred.

In a small percentage of women, the troches can cause irritation in the mouth and/or gums, and occasionally an allergic reac-
tion may occur. Thus I do not prescribe the troches in allergic
persons or asthmatics. Very rarely, women have told me that the
troches increased tooth decay, although this should be possible to
overcome by changing the base used in the troche.

Although theoretically all the hormones in the troches are

designed to be absorbed through the mucous lining of the cheek, directly into the circulation, in many cases it is not possible to avoid swallowing some of the hormones, which will then pass into the intestines and on to the liver. The liver is very efficient at breaking down natural hormones, and thus higher doses of hormones may be needed in the troches to avoid this liver-breakdown effect.

Some women may notice more side-effects from the troches compared to the creams, such as fluid retention, weight gain, breakthrough bleeding and nausea and bloating.

The absorption of the hormones is more rapid from the troches than it is from the creams, and so in women wanting a gentler, more gradual and more sustained effect, I prefer to use the creams. Some doctors prescribe the troches to be cut in halves or quarters, so that they can be taken twice daily, to allow for a more sustained effect. This also reduces the cost of the troches.

The creams can be rubbed into areas where the skin is thinner and well supplied with blood, such as the neck, inner upper arm and inner upper thigh. The creams should not be applied to the breast. The hormones in the cream are well absorbed through the skin directly into the circulation, where they travel to their target tissues to perform their functions before the liver can break them down. This is why many women will find that only small doses of the hormones are needed in the creams, which is desirable for long-term treatment.

To get increased absorption of hormones from the creams, they can be inserted high up into the top of the vagina, with a vaginal applicator. The absorption of hormones from the vagina is very efficient, because of the large surface area of mucosal tissue in the vagina. This increased absorption can be very desirable if natural progesterone is being used to overcome heavy and/or painful menstrual bleeding. The vaginal application of progesterone is also often very successful in women with polycystic ovarian syndrome, who do not ovulate regularly, and thus do not menstruate very often. The use of vaginal progesterone in this way has been shown to overcome over 90 per cent of cases of endometrial hyperplasia (an undesirable overgrowth of the uterine lining).

## When to Use Troches Rather than Creams

- If a woman has found that the creams have been ineffective or inconvenient
- After a hysterectomy, to complement the creams, or as an alternative to the creams
- If the creams cause irritation of the skin and/or vagina, which is rare
- If the creams caused breakthrough bleeding

## When to Use Creams Rather than Troches

- In a high risk woman – such as a woman with varicose veins, a past history of blood clots, liver and/or gall bladder disease, diabetes, Syndrome X, migraine headaches, high blood pressure, heart disease, asthma, allergies, fluid retention or excess weight.
- Women who smoke may be safer using the creams.

## Case History

Lynette came to our hormone clinic complaining of hot flushes, fatigue, unpleasant moods and irritability, and a total loss of interest in sex. She told my colleague that she had not looked forward to the menopause, as her sister and mother had had a rough time going through their menopause. However, she had thought that her symptoms would have come on more gradually than they had, and she was not impressed!

Lynette did not want to take synthetic HRT, as she had read all the adverse publicity about it, and she was seeking a doctor who believed in using the natural types of HRT. She did not want to use patches, as she swam every day in her heated pool and thought that the patches would not stay stuck on her skin. She did not want to take tablets of HRT, as she had a weight problem and suffered with fluid retention.

My colleague correctly started Lynette on a cream containing a daily dose of Triest 2 mg and natural progesterone 50 mg. Lynette returned after three months, saying that she felt much better and had lost some weight without really trying. However, her hot flushes were still bothering her at night and she wanted something stronger.

Before increasing the dose of her HRT, Lynette's doctor decided to get her to take her cream via the vagina – she was told to get a vaginal applicator from the chemist, and insert the cream high up into the vagina last thing at night, when she retired to bed. Theoretically, giving the hormones vaginally may increase the absorption of the hormones into the bloodstream, and this applies especially to the oestrogen called oestradiol. This is because the surface area of the vagina is much larger than that of other areas of skin on the exterior of the body where creams are applied; this is because the vagina has many folds and nooks and crannies. Furthermore, cream applied vaginally cannot, of course, be not rubbed off the skin by clothing. However, remember that if you take oestrogen vaginally you must also take progesterone to avoid over-stimulation of the uterus by unopposed oestrogen.

Lynette used her cream vaginally and returned to the doctor two months later, at which time she told the doctor that her hot flushes were now under control. For Lynette, the simple act of changing the way she used the cream had worked better for her, and she did not need to increase the dose of oestrogen. This is a good little trick to remember for those women wanting to use the smallest dose of hormones in their HRT.

### What Are the Typical Doses Used in Natural HRT?

The doses of hormones used in troches and creams will depend upon what the doctor orders. Thus this type of HRT is far more flexible than brand-name HRT.

Some women will only need very small doses of hormones, and generally speaking it is wise to use the lowesr dose of hormones that will relieve the symptoms.

Let us look at some typical doses that may be used:

| TYPE OF WOMAN | DAILY HORMONE DOSE IN CREAMS | DAILY HORMONE DOSE IN TROCHES |
|---|---|---|
| Women with a uterus | Triest 1 to 4 mg or Oestradiol 0.5 to 2 mg Progesterone 50 to 100 mg DHEA 2 to 5 mg Testosterone 0.5 to 2 mg | Triest 1 to 4 mg or Oestradiol 0.5 to 4mg Progesterone 50 to 400 mg DHEA 5 to 10 mg Testosterone 0.5 to 4 mg |
| Women without a uterus (post-hysterectomy) | Triest 0.5 to 4 mg or Oestradiol 0.5 to 3 mg Progesterone 10 to 50 mg DHEA 2 to 5 mg Testosterone 0.5 to 2 mg | Triest 1 to 4 mg or Oestradiol 0.5 to 4 mg Progesterone 25 to 100 mg DHEA 5 tp 10 mg Testosterone 0.5 to 4 mg |

These doses are to give you a 'ballpark figure' only, as the doses that you may require will need to be worked out by your own doctor after blood and/or saliva tests are done. Everyone is a unique case, and in women with risk factors such as liver/gall bladder disease, high blood pressure, a past history of blood clots or other risk factors, doctors will often prescribe smaller doses than those in the Table above.

In males receiving treatment for male menopause (andropause), some typical doses that may be used are:

| HORMONE | DAILY HORMONE DOSE IN CREAMS | DAILY HORMONE DOSE IN TROCHES |
|---------|------------------------------|-------------------------------|
| DHEA | 5 to 20 mg | 10 to 50 mg |
| Testosterone | 2 to 5 mg | 10 to 20 mg |

Generally speaking, as with women, doctors will use the lowest doses of hormones necessary to relieve the symptoms of the male menopause. Excessive doses of testosterone can lead to an elevation of cholesterol and an increased risk of prostate cancer.

### Are Hormone Patches a Good Form of HRT?

Hormone patches were a great breakthrough for women when they first arrived on the scene over a decade ago. This was because the patch was suitable for women who needed oestrogen but could not tolerate it orally because it aggravated pre-existing medical problems such as liver/gall bladder disease, migraines, varicose veins or hypertension. Patches can also be used by smokers and people with diabetes, or women with high triglyceride levels in their blood.

The patch is adhesive, and delivers oestradiol at a controlled rate through the skin directly into the bloodstream. Thus it bypasses the liver, and much smaller doses of hormones can be used in the patches. The patch is applied to dry clean skin on the buttocks, thighs or abdomen, and is replaced with a new patch once or twice a week. Some women become allergic to the adhesive in the patch, which causes skin irritation and redness. If skin irritation becomes bothersome, transdermal hormone creams can be used instead of the patches. Some women find that the patch does not stick well to the skin if they wear it in the shower or bath, so you can take it off, before showering, and reapply the patch once your skin is dry.

Other women find that if they live in a hot climate, or swim regularly, the patch does not stay on, in which case hormone creams may be more practical and effective.

The first transdermal oestrogen patch was approved for use by the US Food and Drug Administration in the 1980s. Since this time, many types of patches have come onto the market, so that a large variety of strengths is now available. There is also a combination patch, which contains oestradiol and synthetic progestogen. The combination patch can be used in women who still have a uterus, and thus need to take some form of progesterone with their oestrogen. For women who do not want to take progesterone orally, they can now take it in the patch. Although the combination patch contains synthetic progesterone, because the doses of hormones in the patch are so low, there are generally very few side-effects, if any. Most women using the combination patch do not have any periods, which is a welcome relief.

The hormone patches are just as effective as the oral forms of HRT in relieving the symptoms of the menopause and in reducing osteoporosis.

For the brand names and doses of the different patches, see the Table on page 239.

**Suggested Application Sites of Estraderm Patches**

Estraderm 25

Estraderm 50

Estraderm 100

1 & 2 First Week
3 & 4 Second Week
1 & 2 Third Week etc

# Chapter 6

# What are the Super Hormones?

The term 'Super Hormones' has been used to describe a group of **anti-ageing hormones**. This group of hormones is increasingly used to rejuvenate the endocrine system in middle-aged and older persons.

The natural hormones that belong to this group are:

- Pregnenolone
- DHEA
- Growth Hormone
- Testosterone
- Melatonin

Some people would also consider the three natural oestrogens and progesterone as part of the Super Hormone group, as they can definitely exert anti-ageing effects.

These hormones are usually given in the form of lozenges, capsules, sub-lingual drops or creams, although Growth Hormone is only effective if injected.

The Super Hormones can make a huge difference to men and women in their forties, fifties and beyond, who suffer with chronic fatigue, insomnia, depression, poor memory, and aches and pains (fibromyalgia). These hormones require a doctor's prescription. Homoeopathic doses or brands of Super Hormones are ineffective.

### DHEA – An Anti-ageing Hormone

DHEA stands for De-hydro-epi-androsterone and is a hormone made in both sexes; however DHEA was not identified as a sex hormone in women until the late 1950s.

DHEA is a natural hormone produced mainly by the adrenal glands. Small quantities are also made in the brain, testicles and ovaries. The pituitary hormone called ACTH stimulates the production of DHEA from the adrenal glands.

In men, DHEA is present in much greater amounts than testosterone. Like pregnenolone, DHEA can be called a 'mother hormone' as it can be converted in the body into other steroid hormones. The body's production of DHEA peaks at a young age (around 25), and declines steadily after this age. The amounts of DHEA in the saliva are only 0.1 per cent of its concentration in the blood.

DHEA is present in the body in two forms:

1. DHEA, which is the active hormone in the body
2. DHEA–S (sulphate), which is inactive in the body.

The brain contains much higher amounts of DHEA than any other hormone, and the bloodstream contains higher levels of the inactive DHEA–S. Interestingly, women have higher levels of active DHEA in their brain than men!

The DHEA–S acts as a reserve supply, which releases active DHEA to the body tissues and organs as required.

*Factors that Increase DHEA Production in the Body*

- puberty
- lactation
- pregnancy
- exercise
- meditation

*Factors that Decrease DHEA Production in the Body*

- adrenal gland dysfunction, or disease
- ageing
- prolonged stress or illness
- auto-immune diseases
- high alcohol intake or heavy smoking
- underactive thyroid gland
- some types of depressive illness
- certain types of medications such as some anti-epilepsy drugs, the contraceptive pill, some cholesterol lowering drugs, cimetidine and ketoconazole.

In the US many people take DHEA as an anti-ageing hormone. Some researchers consider that DHEA is able to help offset the effects of ageing. DHEA is also available as a nutritional supplement in the US, where it is easily obtained from health food stores without a prescription. In Australia, DHEA is only available with a doctor's prescription, and is generally prescribed for chronic fatigue syndrome/ME and/or adrenal gland exhaustion.

The blood and/or salivary levels of DHEA should be measured before deciding if DHEA replacement is needed. If you decide to stay on DHEA, your doctor should do a blood or saliva test every few months, to ensure that the level of DHEA does not become excessive.

DHEA should not be used in patients who have hormone sensitive cancers, or who have excess male hormones.

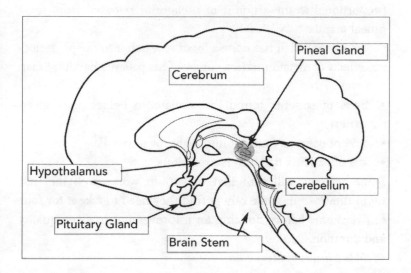

## Can Melatonin Help?

The hormone melatonin is made in the pineal gland, which is buried deep in the brain.

In the pineal gland, the amino acid tryptophan is converted to serotonin, then to N-acetyl serotonin, and then methylated to produce melatonin. The chemical name for melatonin is 5-methoxyl-N-acetyl-tryptamine.

Melatonin is involved in inducing REM sleep, which is the phase of deep sleep during which dreams occur. Daylight inhibits the production of melatonin, and darkness stimulates the production of melatonin. Beginning at sunset and continuing throughout the night, the pineal gland secretes melatonin; peak levels are reached between 2 and 4 a.m.

Melatonin has been generally used as a hormone to promote a deep and restful natural sleeping pattern. It certainly is a welcome alternative to sleeping pills, and may help menopausal women, in whom insomnia is a common complaint. Researchers have found that the quality of sleep among older people is proportional to the amount of melatonin released from their pineal glands.

Dr Ray Sahelian has done a lot of research into the physiological effects of melatonin. In a survey of his patients he found that:

- 80% of patients found that melatonin helped their sleep patterns
- 15% of patients found it ineffective or too weak
- 5% of patients had adverse reactions.

Some patients will find that melatonin works well the first night they take it, while others find they need to take it for four to five nights before noticing an improvement in sleep quality and duration.

*Possible Benefits of Melatonin*

- improved sleep
- relief of jetlag-induced insomnia
- improvement of sleep and biorhythms in shift workers.

## MELATONIN AND LIFESPAN

The researcher Dr Pierpaoli has discovered that melatonin increased the lifespan of male mice by 20 per cent. This could be because of the antioxidant properties of melatonin. Melatonin is able to scavenge free radicals, and is also efficient in preventing free radical-induced damage.

The researcher Hardeland has found that melatonin was a more effective antioxidant than vitamins C and E, although these vitamins work in different ways, and are still vital for health.

The researcher Maestroni has observed a link between the function of the thymus gland and melatonin. He found that melatonin promotes the manufacture of T-lymphocytes in those with a dysfunctional immune system. Melatonin appears to have some ability to support the thymus gland, increase interferon production and augment anti-cancer factors.

Another interesting role of melatonin that is worthy of more research is its observed inhibitory effect on some types of cancer cells. The researcher Hill has found that melatonin exerts a direct, lethal action on oestrogen-sensitive breast cancer cells in the laboratory. Thus melatonin could possibly augment the anti-cancer effects of other drugs, such as tamoxifen. Wilson conducted an interesting experiment, where he exposed human breast cancer cells to melatonin and then exposed these same cells to the drug tamoxifen. The pre-exposure with melatonin increased the inhibitory effects of tamoxifen on the cancer cells.

For those with some types of immune dysfunction, melatonin is worth considering as a restorative substance that may improve the quantity and quality of life.

## SIDE-EFFECTS OF MELATONIN

Reported side-effects from melatonin are related to the doses used, and are infrequent in those using less than 3 mg of melatonin daily. The dose can easily be reduced down to 1 mg in those who cannot tolerate 3 mg.

*Reported Side-effects*

- fatigue and a 'hangover' feeling the following morning (15% of users)
- unpleasant dreams (5% of users)
- headache (2% of users)
- reduced sex drive (2% of users)
- depression with long-term use (2% of users)

Side-effects are not permanent, and cease quickly after stopping melatonin. There have been no reports of addiction to melatonin, and there are usually no withdrawal symptoms after ceasing it.

## WHEN SHOULD MELATONIN NOT BE USED?

- Melatonin is a stimulant of the immune system, and as such should not be used by people suffering auto-immune diseases such as Lupus (SLE), or cancers of the white blood cells such as lymphoma or leukaemia.
- Pregnant or breastfeeding women should avoid melatonin until further research of its safety during these states has been done.
- Caution should be used if the patient is taking anti-depressant drugs, as these drugs may already increase melatonin levels.
- Those with problems of the adrenal glands, or diabetes, should consult their endocrinologist before trying melatonin.

## DOSES OF MELATONIN

Melatonin is generally prescribed in doses of 1 to 3 mg. It is taken at sunset.

It is available only on a doctor's prescription and comes as sublingual drops or troches.

# Chapter 7

# Can Hormones Help Your Sex Life?

I am consulted by many women about their loss of sex drive and sexual enjoyment during the peri-menopausal years. They often ask for help, saying that it is their partner who has requested that they seek help due to the disparity in their sex drives. They are often a little embarrassed or shy when they begin to talk about these matters. Many are very relieved to be able to talk with a female doctor about these sensitive issues.

## Factors that Can Impair Your Sex Life

- reduction of sex hormone production in the body as we age
- fear of pregnancy. During the peri-menopause, fertility can be unpredictable. Once the menopause is diagnosed conclusively by the finding of persistently elevated FSH levels, the fear of unwanted pregnancy is eliminated, and this can have a positive effect on your sex life. This was an observation that was very obvious when I worked in a missionary hospital in India during the 1980s.
- the oral contraceptive pill often reduces libido because it reduces the amounts of free sex hormones in the body
- general health – medical problems such as diabetes, heart disease, thyroid dysfunction, chronic fatigue and anaemia may reduce libido. Women who have been treated for cancer

with chemotherapy or radiotherapy will be suffering side-effects from these treatments and will also have to cope with the effects of a chemically-induced premature menopause.

- problems with your relationship, which are most commonly due to difficulties in communication and lack of understanding of the changing sexual needs that may occur during the menopause. If these are important issues for you, please seek help for both yourself and your partner from a professional counsellor or sex therapist.
- physical changes such as vaginal dryness, reduction in elasticity of the vagina, shrinkage of the vagina and clitoris, pelvic pain during intercourse, loss of pelvic floor muscle tone and urinary incontinence
- problems with your body image, including physical changes in the vulva, loss of pubic hair, vaginal prolapse, excess weight, a change in body odour and loss of body tone
- hot flushes, profuse sweating and disturbed sleep, may be off-putting to a close relationship in bed
- depression and stress may adversely affect your desire for, and enjoyment of, sex
- certain medications may reduce libido either slightly or dramatically, such as – oral oestrogens and progestogens (as found in conventional HRT and the oral contraceptive pill), anti-male hormones such as cyproterone acetate and spironolactone, beta-blockers, cholesterol-lowering medication, some anti-depressants, sedatives and drugs that interfere with acid production by the stomach ($H_2$ antagonists).

The hormones that have the greatest influence upon our sex drive are oestrogen and testosterone. In women troubled by a low libido it is important to do a blood test to check the levels of these hormones. If they are found to be very low, or at the lower limit of the normal range, replacement with the deficient hormone can be very effective.

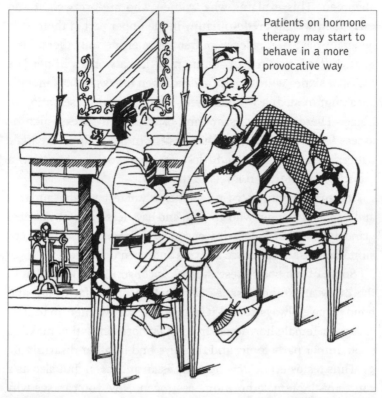

Patients on hormone therapy may start to behave in a more provocative way

The hormone testosterone is a very important hormone in women, and has the biggest effect upon increasing the sex drive.

Parts of the Body that Manufacture Testosterone

- the adrenal glands (approximately 25% of the total testosterone)
- the ovaries (approximately 25% of the total testosterone)
- the fat tissue (approximately 50% of the total testosterone)

In the fat tissue, testosterone is produced from the hormone called androstenedione. Most of this conversion occurs in the fat tissue in the upper part of the body, such as in the trunk and abdomen. This explains why women who are overweight and carry their weight predominantly in the upper part of their body generally have higher levels of free testosterone and other androgens. Indeed, it is not uncommon to find a woman in her late fifties or sixties with a high free androgen index (FAI). Generally speaking, in such a woman there is often good preservation of libido. There may be symptoms of androgen excess such as excess facial/body hair, and hair loss from the scalp in the male pattern of baldness. Weight loss in such women results in a reduction of androgen levels in the body.

It is more common to find a deficiency of testosterone and free androgens in women who are thin and have less body fat. Adrenal gland dysfunction, low body weight and the menopause can occur simultaneously to produce a severe androgen deficiency.

Some of the body's testosterone is converted to oestrogen in the ovary and other tissues such as the brain, fat tissue and bone. I have always found it interesting that women manufacture their female hormones from male hormones; this makes a good dinner party topic, and the guys find it rather disarming!

Thus testosterone acts not only as an androgen, but also as a source of the female hormone oestrogen. Now you can see why thin women often have much lower levels of testosterone and oestrogen during the peri-menopausal years, compared to women with more body fat.

The vast majority of the testosterone in the bloodstream is bound to proteins such as Sex Hormone Binding Globulin (SHBG) and albumin, and only 1 per cent of the total testosterone is not bound to protein. This 1 per cent is called free testosterone, and is the active hormone in the body. The hormone that is bound to proteins is unavailable to act on the tissues, and is thus inactive.

The amount of SHBG in the body is important, as when high

levels of SHBG are present there will be fewer free androgens to act on the tissues. Low levels of SHBG will result in higher amounts of free androgens to be available to the body. When the hormone levels in women with a low libido are evaluated, attention needs to be paid to the levels of SHBG, the total testosterone and the levels of the free male hormones (Free Androgen Index or FAI). The measurement of total testosterone levels alone is inadequate to assess the overall impact of the hormone levels upon libido.

**What Are the Factors that Influence the Level of SHBG in the Body?**

*Factors that Lower SHBG Levels*

- weight excess, especially associated with Syndrome X
- a diet high in sugar and refined carbohydrate and hydrogenated fats
- Polycystic Ovarian Syndrome (PCOS)
- treatment with the HRT tablet called Tibolone
- treatment with cortisone
- growth hormone
- treatment with testosterone
- ageing

*Factors that Increase SHBG Levels*

- oestrogen tablets – in HRT or the contraceptive pill
- high doses of oestrogen in HRT
- treatment with thyroid hormone tablets
- pregnancy

*Blood Tests Required to Evaluate the Overall Hormone Status of a Woman Troubled by Low Libido*

- FSH and oestrogen and progesterone levels
- Total testosterone levels – levels in the lower part of the normal range are not considered ideal for a good libido
- The Free Androgen Index (FAI) evaluates the amount of free testosterone and other androgens that are unbound to proteins and are active in the body. The normal range for FAI

is generally reported by most laboratories as 0.1 to 8.0. However, if the FAI is less than 3 in a patient who complains of sexual dysfunction, then replacement with testosterone and/or DHEA is likely to be of great benefit. Indeed, it may be dramatically beneficial and greatly improve not only the sex life, but overall physical and mental well-being.

While women are receiving hormone replacement therapy, and especially testosterone therapy to treat their sexual problems, it is important to measure the levels of these hormones in blood or saliva tests. Physicians do not want to produce extremely high levels of hormones, as the phenomena of tachyphylaxis may occur – this is where a woman becomes accustomed to very high levels of hormones such as oestrogen and testosterone in her body, and normal levels of hormones no longer work. The aim of treatment is to restore the levels of testosterone into the middle of the normal range, and not above upper limits. In women using hormone implants, before another implant is inserted, it is important to prove that a new implant is really needed by checking the blood levels of the relevant hormone.

It is now recognized formally that a state of male hormone (androgen) deficiency may exist in women. The Princeton Consensus Statement defines female androgen-deficiency syndrome as follows:

- a diminished sense of well-being, unpleasant moods and reduced motivation
- frequent and persistent fatigue for which no other cause is evident
- impaired sexual function – including reduced sex drive and reduced sexual pleasure and response
- possible bone loss and decreased muscle strength
- a reduction in mental efficiency.

I have also found that fibromyalgia is a common complaint in those with reduced androgen levels in the body.

The loss of sex hormone-production in the body can cause changes in the pelvic organs such as:

- thinning of the pubic hair
- shrinkage and loss of sensitivity of the vulva and clitoris – it may become increasingly difficult to orgasm
- weakening of the support of the vaginal wall
- an increase in vaginal prolapse
- dryness and thinning of the vaginal lining and vulva – this may make sexual intercourse uncomfortable and even impossible
- shrinkage of the vagina – this may make penetration painful
- a reduced acidity in the vagina, which increases the chances of infection and inflammation
- loss of fat from the lips of the vaginal opening (the vulva)
- unpleasant sensations in the vulva and clitoris, such as stinging, burning and/or a crawling feeling. It may feel as if ants are biting the area, and there may be a desire to scratch. If the clitoris or vulva is touched, this may produce unpleasant sensations. These symptoms can be misinterpreted as infection, and many women do not realize that hormone deficiency can cause these problems.
- bladder dysfunction with symptoms of urinary frequency, urgency and burning. Bladder infections may occur.

In women with an early menopause, or after hysterectomy, problems with low libido are common, and hormonal therapy is worth considering. Natural oestrogen and/or testosterone can be given in small doses, and gradually increased, until sex drive and sexual enjoyment are restored. Testosterone increases sex drive and the sensitivity and size of the clitoris, which will often help those women who have lost the ability to orgasm. Oestrogen makes the breasts fuller and rounder, and increases nipple sensitivity and lubrication of the vagina and vulva.

DHEA can increase libido, probably because it acts like a weaker form of testosterone. DHEA is a precursor of pheromones in some animals, and probably in humans as well. Pheromones are hormones which attract sexual partners! During orgasm the amount of DHEA in the brain increases.

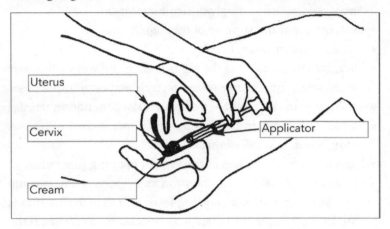

Uterus

Cervix

Applicator

Cream

## How Hormones Can Be Administered to Increase Sex Drive and Enjoyment

I have found that the most effective way to take libido-enhancing hormones is in the form of troches (lozenges), creams and/or injections.

### OESTROGEN INJECTIONS

Oestrogen injections can be given into the fat of the buttocks. The injection will give a boost of oestrogen that will last for three to six weeks. These injections are relatively potent and can provide a quick effect, which can be desirable if you want to start a sexual relationship quickly after a long period of no HRT. The injections **quickly** restore the sex drive, and lubrication of the vagina and vulva, and increase the size and sensitivity of the breasts.

Injections are best used only as a temporary measure, as if they were to be used regularly on a long-term basis they may provide excess levels of oestrogen, which could theoretically increase the risk of breast cancer. Nevertheless, the injections have a role for a woman who has been without any hormones in her body for several months, and who finds herself needing emergency HRT to start or rejuvenate her sexual relationships.

## TABLETS

Tablet forms of HRT are not as effective at boosting sex drive, and may not be a safe solution to be used on a long-term basis. One of the reasons why tablet (oral) forms of HRT are not as effective in boosting sex drive and pleasure is that they induce the liver to make extra amounts of the protein called Sex Hormone Binding Globulin (SHBG). SHBG binds the sex hormones so that they are not available to the cells, and thus they remain inactive. The more SHBG that is present in your bloodstream, the less will be the amount of free hormones available to work on your cells. Thus although you may be taking large doses of hormones in tablets, the hormones are being inactivated by the SHBG. One exception here is the synthetic hormone tablet called Tibolone, which lowers SHBG and can be effective in increasing libido.

Because the small amount of hormones absorbed from creams does not increase the production of SHBG in the liver, much smaller doses of hormones are effective at boosting the sex drive.

## HORMONE PATCHES

Hormone patches containing oestrogen and synthetic progesterone may have a slight effect in boosting libido; however for women with a very low sex drive, or for women with vaginal dryness and discomfort, the patches by themselves will often be inadequate. In the near future a patch containing testosterone will be available for women, although I think the creams are more practical and effective, especially as you can use them locally on the vulva and clitoris.

## TESTOSTERONE IMPLANTS

Testosterone can be given in the form of an implant; however some women will find this too strong, and notice an increase in facial hair and/or acne, and weight gain. Generally 50 to 100 mg of testosterone is given in the implant, and it lasts from three to six months.

## TESTOSTERONE INJECTIONS

Some women are given testosterone injections in doses from 50 to 100 mg intramuscularly, every four to six weeks. These can be very effective and give you a very strong libido, which may be difficult to control! Indeed, some husbands complain that they have been worn out and come seeking help themselves, merely to keep up with the increased demand for sex from their newly energized partner! The injections are not ideal in the long term, as the blood levels of testosterone tend to go from too high to too low, and the dosage is too hard to control.

Testosterone can also be given orally, in the form of testosterone undecanoate tablets in a dose of 40 mg daily; however, these pass through the liver and may exert adverse metabolic changes, as well as weight gain.

The synthetic HRT tablet called Tibolone exerts an androgenic effect in the body, and reduces the levels of SHBG. In a significant percentage of users, Tibolone will improve the sex life.

## CREAMS

Creams containing natural hormones can exert a satisfactory long-term effect in boosting libido and sexual satisfaction in women of all ages. Because the doses of hormones needed in the creams are low, the creams are safer than tablets.

To increase the sex drive, the best combination of natural hormones mixed together in *one* cream is:

- Oestrogen in the form of oestradiol (0.5 to 2 mg)
- Progesterone (20 to 100 mg)
- Testosterone and/or DHEA (0.5 to 2 mg)

This cream can be applied to the lips of the vulva and the clitoris every night. The cream is best applied when you are ready to go to sleep, *after* sex and after emptying your bladder. Part of the cream can also be inserted into the vagina with an applicator. Your doctor will tell you how much cream to insert into the vagina, and how much to massage into the vulva. I usually tell my patients to insert one-third of the dose into the vagina, and the other two-thirds on the vulval area.

If the clitoris has shrunk and/or is tender, irritated or very fragile, the cream can be massaged into the clitoris every night. This usually overcomes all these problems.

Creams containing a mixture of the above natural hormones will restore and rejuvenate the vagina, vulva and clitoris.

*Benefits of Creams on Your Sex Life*
- a reduction in vaginal dryness and discomfort during sex
- an increase in the sensitivity of the vulva, clitoris and vagina
- a reduction of shrinkage of the vagina
- the restoration of the ability to have orgasms
- a reduction in bladder problems such as infection, incontinence and urgency
- an increase in sex drive

The hormones in the cream are absorbed into the cells of the vagina and vulva, and thus exert a local restorative effect. There are large numbers of hormone receptors in the vulva and vagina, and thus the local effect of these hormones is much more predominant than any other effects upon the body. This means that using creams will produce less chance of general side-effects compared to hormone tablets, implants or injections.

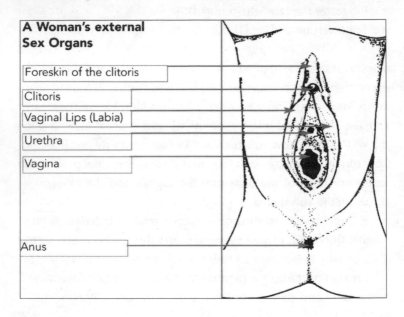

### A Woman's external Sex Organs

- Foreskin of the clitoris
- Clitoris
- Vaginal Lips (Labia)
- Urethra
- Vagina
- Anus

There will be some absorption of the hormones from the vaginal cream into the bloodstream, which will make a woman feel more feminine and desirable. Women who do not want to absorb significant amounts of hormones into their bloodstream will need to avoid inserting the cream into the vagina, and use the cream on the vulva and clitoris only. For many women, especially as they get older, this is all they need to do to restore their sex life.

### Other Therapies to Improve the Sex Life

- Phytoestrogens – found in some foods such as soybeans, alfalfa sprouts and whole flaxseed – can produce a worthwhile increase in libido, and improve the sex life during the menopause.
- Pelvic floor exercises are very effective at improving vaginal tone and reducing vaginal prolapse – they are best taught by a physiotherapist and I also recommend the little book called *Woman's Waterworks* by Pauline Chiarelli.
- Vaginal lubricants such as KY jelly, which do not contain any hormones, may be helpful during sex.
- Specific gels can be applied to the vulva and clitoris, and may enable or enhance orgasms. There are various brands available and they usually contain a mixture of non-hormonal ingredients such as: L-ornithine, L-arginine, menthol crystals, peppermint oil, lecithin, grapefruit seed extract, and ginseng and gingko biloba. Some women find that they work quite well, while others find them unsatisfactory, or even totally useless.

### What About Your Partner?

It is not uncommon that when a patient returns to see me for a follow-up consultation, she will say, 'Well, my hormones are working now, but my partner needs some help to keep up with me!' Many men are reluctant to seek help for sexual problems such as loss of libido and erectile dysfunction, as they are embarrassed or ashamed to talk about them. For the reluctant partner, I often suggest that we start by having some blood tests done. I then give the woman a request form for her partner, so that he can go to a local pathology laboratory with the request form, and have his blood taken.

*Blood Tests for the Male with Possible Hormone Problems*
- total serum testosterone (and salivary testosterone)
- free testosterone

- DHEA-S and salivary DHEA
- Free Androgen Index (FAI)
- Sex Hormone Binding Globulin (SHBG)

If his results indicate low levels of male hormones, the next step is to refer the male to a urologist, who will do a full check-up of the prostate gland. This is because undiagnosed problems with the prostate gland, such as prostate enlargement or prostate cancer, can be aggravated by androgen therapy. If the urologist gives the patient a clear result, then some natural hormone replacement can be used to restore his hormone levels back to normal amounts. The best hormones for men to increase their libido are natural testosterone **and** DHEA, which can be prescribed in the form of a troche or cream.

*Typical Doses of HRT for Men*
- Testosterone: 5 to 10 mg daily
- DHEA: 20 mg daily

I do not recommend tablets or injections of testosterone, as these are very potent and much more likely to produce side-effects such as stimulation of the prostate gland, weight gain and elevated cholesterol levels. With the creams and/or troches the doses of hormones can easily be reduced, and can be adjusted over time so that the smallest possible dose can be used to produce good results.

Natural testosterone and/or DHEA can also produce a worthwhile improvement in moods, confidence, energy levels and muscle strength. They can also help to reduce aches and pains.

For erectile problems, Viagra is excellent; however it does not have any hormonal effect and will not directly increase the libido. Viagra can make an impotent man potent again, however it will not always make his desire or inclination any greater.

For men who suffer with premature ejaculation associated with depression and/or anxiety, the use of the modern anti-depressant drugs known as Selective Serotonin Re-uptake Inhibitors (SSRIs) can produce a cure.

## Case History

Joanne came to see me on a bus all the way from Lightening Ridge, a small opal-mining town in Northwestern New South Wales, as she had trouble getting help for her menopausal problems in her home town. She had been prescribed combined oral HRT but was not getting the relief she had hoped for. She complained of depression and weight gain in the abdominal area, and fatigue, and said that she felt 'out of sorts'. I asked her what she had told her local doctor and she said, 'Well, I told him that I have lost all my libidoooo!' Perhaps her doctor had not understood her particular way of saying 'libidoooo!'

After a few giggles, we decided that she definitely needed to do something about her 'libidoooo', particularly as her husband was some years younger than she and was having almost as much difficulty accepting the changes her body was going through as she was herself.

Joanne suffered with vaginal dryness and discomfort and had lost the ability to orgasm, which worried her considerably. On examination, her vaginal tissue looked thin and dry, and her clitoris had shrunk. We decided that she would be best to stop the hormone tablets, as they were probably contributing to her weight gain and had not helped with her sexual problems.

The results of her blood tests showed low levels of oestradiol, low FAI and elevated SHBG. No wonder she had no libidoooo!

I prescribed a hormonal cream containing a mixture of oestradiol (2 mg), progesterone (40 mg) and testosterone (2 mg). Joanne was told to massage this cream into her vulva and clitoral area every day. The best time for her to do this was *after* sex and after emptying her bladder, last thing at night when she was ready to sleep.

I also prescribed for her the combined patch containing oestrogen and progestogen to balance the effect of the local creams.

Well, after six weeks I received a letter from a very grateful Joanne, telling me that her libidoooo was now working very well and she was able to enjoy sexual relations with her husband once again. She had also lost weight and was no longer bloated or tired.

Yes, Joanne was swinging from the chandeliers!

# Chapter 8

# Weight Control During and
# After the Menopause

Weight gain is a very common complaint in peri-menopausal women. Indeed, many women who have never had a problem with their weight, arrive at the menopause and then suddenly seem to pile it on for no apparent reason. Yes, 'apparent' is the word, because there are often *hidden problems* with the metabolism that are responsible for this weight gain.

*Unwanted weight gain at menopause is most commonly due to one or a combination of the following factors:*
- Syndrome X – the chemical imbalance that makes your metabolism store fat
- liver dysfunction – the liver stops burning fat efficiently, and indeed you may develop a fatty liver, infiltrated with unhealthy fat. In such cases, unless liver function can be improved, it is impossible to lose weight.
- underactivity of the thyroid gland, which causes a slowing down of the metabolic rate
- inappropriate hormone replacement therapy with oral forms of potent hormones
- excessive doses of HRT, especially testosterone

- stress eating to cope with anxiety, boredom and/or depression
- lack of exercise in women who have medical problems, or not enough time for themselves.

*The most common cause of excessive weight gain during and after the menopause is Syndrome X!*

## SYNDROME X

For those who battle with their weight, Syndrome X is a fascinating subject and explains the difficulty many menopausal women have in controlling their weight as they get older.

### HOW DOES SYNDROME X DEVELOP IN THE BODY?

Syndrome X begins with the phenomenon of insulin resistance, which means that the body gradually becomes resistant to the effect of its own insulin. The body compensates for this by producing more and more insulin, resulting in excess levels of insulin in the blood. Insulin is the hormone that is produced by the pancreas to control the metabolism of sugar and fat in the body.

High levels of insulin are undesirable because:

- *Insulin is a fat storing hormone* – insulin converts excess dietary carbohydrates into body fat.
- *Insulin suppresses the levels of the fat-burning hormones in your body* – thus it stops you from burning body fat for energy. Thus, high levels of insulin not only make you fat, they make sure that you stay fat – yes, Syndrome X is a double-edged sword!
- *High insulin levels make you very hungry* – insulin stimulates the appetite, and makes you crave carbohydrates such as bread, biscuits, cakes, muffins, snack foods, pasta, noodles, rice, grains, cereals and sugar. The high levels of insulin will turn these carbohydrates into body fat, which explains why you can become very overweight even on a fat-free diet!

No wonder that those with Syndrome X find themselves trapped in a metabolic nightmare, and often believe it is their weak will power that is to blame. Well, stop feeling guilty! Syndrome X is not a psychological problem; it is a chemical imbalance that redirects your metabolism into fat-storing.

High levels of insulin can be very toxic and may result in other health problems such as:

- high levels of the bad LDL cholesterol
- low levels of the good HDL cholesterol
- high levels of the fat triglycerides
- increased plaque-formation in the arteries
- fluid-retention
- elevated blood pressure
- unstable blood sugar levels, which can lead to type 2 diabetes.

Syndrome X can be compared to an iceberg – all you see are the symptoms above the surface, but the cause of Syndrome X, namely insulin imbalance, remains hidden. Unless we correct the insulin imbalance, it is impossible to lose weight.

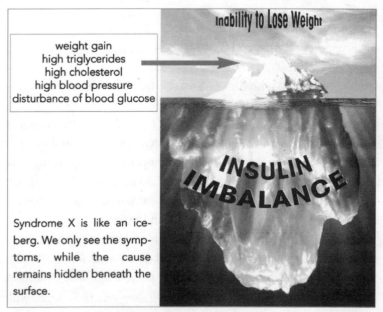

Inability to Lose Weight

weight gain
high triglycerides
high cholesterol
high blood pressure
disturbance of blood glucose

INSULIN IMBALANCE

Syndrome X is like an iceberg. We only see the symptoms, while the cause remains hidden beneath the surface.

## HEART DISEASE

The metabolic problems caused by Syndrome X are risk factors for cardiovascular disease, especially if you have several of them. Few women think that they will die of cardiovascular disease; the fact is it's their number one killer. Heart disease is by far the leading cause of death among women. I have found that the biggest fear of most women is of breast cancer, and many women believe that breast cancer is the most common cause of death. This is not true. Cardiovascular diseases such as heart disease, blood clots and strokes are responsible for nearly half of all female deaths. A woman has nearly a 25 per cent risk of dying from heart attack. Following a heart attack, women are more likely than men to have another. Women are twice as likely as men to die within six weeks of a heart attack, and are less likely to survive over the long term.

The risk of heart attack in women is in stark contrast to the much lower risk of her dying from other causes:

- Breast cancer – 4%
- Bone fractures – 2.5%
- Cancers of the reproductive tract – 2%

For every woman who dies of breast cancer, five die of cardiovascular disease.

In pre-menopausal women, the risk of cardiovascular disease is low. We know that women begin to catch up to men in their risk status after they pass through the menopause. The Framingham study indicated that the menopause, in itself, is a major risk factor for heart disease; indeed, it appeared to triple the risk. It appears that the loss of our natural oestrogen and progesterone has a contributory effect towards diseases of the blood vessels and heart.

We can greatly offset this loss of hormonal protection by controlling the problem of Syndrome X, which is a powerful predictor of cardiovascular disease.

## HOW CAN YOU OVERCOME SYNDROME X?

The most scientific way to overcome Syndrome X is to treat the *cause* – namely, to lower the excessive insulin levels in the body. We can achieve this by changing the way we eat, so that we do not continually stimulate the production of excess insulin in our body.

My book, *Can't Lose Weight? You could have Syndrome X* provides a 12-week eating plan to lower insulin levels, and thus redirect your metabolism from fat-storing into fat-burning.

## Lowering Insulin Levels

- **Eat first-class proteins three times a day**, and also if you get hungry between meals.

  Good sources of first class protein are:

  Lean fresh red and white meats

  Seafood – all types are suitable

  Eggs – preferably organic

  Poultry – preferably organic

  Some cheeses – the best cheeses for weight-watchers are Parmesan, feta, ricotta and low-fat cottage cheese

  Whey protein powder – available at health food shops

  Combining nuts, seeds and legumes (beans, peas, lentils) at the **same** meal

- **Be careful with Carbohydrates**

  All carbohydrates are converted to sugar (glucose) in the body, and thus have the potential to stimulate increased insulin levels. Most people with Syndrome X eat too much carbohydrate, and will not be able to lose weight easily unless they reduce the amount of carbohydrate in their daily diet. Many people have a diet that is loaded with carbohydrates – just think about it! You start the day with cereal and toast, then have a sandwich for lunch, and more bread, pasta, noodles and desserts at night. This style of eating will ensure that your insulin levels stay high all day, and keep you in the fat-storing zone.

Avoid refined carbohydrates such as sugar, refined flours and foods with added sugar. Check food labels for added or hidden sugars such as maltodextrin, dextrin and high fructose corn syrup.

The best carbohydrates are unrefined and high in fibre, and include things such as muesli with no added sugar, legumes, unprocessed grains and unprocessed wholegrain breads. These types of carbohydrates are slowly absorbed from the gut, and thus do not abruptly raise blood sugar levels – they are known as low Glycaemic Index (GI) carbohydrates.

In those people who have been overweight for years and who find it very difficult to lose weight, it can be necessary to avoid most carbohydrates for several months. If this is not done, the high insulin levels will not come down, and thus fat-burning cannot commence.

Those women who find it impossible to lose weight often have such a sluggish metabolism that we can call them 'metabolically resistant'. To enable these women to begin to lose weight, it is necessary to exclude *all* added sugar, *all* grains (wheat, rye, barley, oats, corn, rice etc), and *all* foods made from grains (e.g. bread, pasta, biscuits, crackers, cereals, noodles, cakes, puddings, etc.) for two to six months. They can have legumes, raw nuts and seeds, but *no* grains until they have lost a significant amount of weight. This 'no grain, no sugar'diet will work for those who have found it impossible to lose weight. The diet is similar to the way that cavemen used to eat: they did not have grains or added sugar, and their bodies consisted of bone and muscle and very little fat.

Very low-carbohydrate diets, containing less then 40 grams of carbohydrate daily, are called *ketogenic* diets, and are very effective for metabolically-resistant people.

If you decide to follow a ketogenic diet, you should be supervised by a naturopath or doctor. For more information you can visit www.weightcontroldoctor.com

- **Eat plenty of vegetables, fruits and other plant foods**

  I encourage you to increase the amount of plant foods such as vegetables, fruits, raw seeds and nuts, and legumes (beans, peas and lentils) in your daily diet. These foods contain plant hormones known as phytoestrogens, which are known to reduce the risk of many types of cancer. Many of the currently popular high-protein weight-loss diets do not contain enough plant food, because of paranoia about carbohydrates. While it may be necessary to reduce plant carbohydrates for several months in order for those with Syndrome X to start losing weight, in the long term it is vital to consume plenty of plant foods to reduce the risk of cancer as you get older. Plant foods are also essential for a healthy liver and immune system, and most people do not get enough vegetables, fruits and legumes in their daily diet. Many of my overweight patients tell me that they only eat salads during the summer, if at all. No wonder they have a sluggish liver that does not burn fat efficiently! If you want to control your weight easily, you need to eat salads every day.

  Fruits and vegetables do contain carbohydrates, but because their carbohydrates are combined with vitamins, minerals and fibre, they are more easily handled by the body. Fruits contain the sugar known as fructose, which does not spike insulin levels very much compared to the sugars sucrose and glucose. Generally, three to four pieces of fruit can be eaten daily. The best fruits for weight loss are: all citrus, apples, persimmons, pineapples and berries of all varieties.

- **Eat the healthy fats**

  It is important to have an adequate intake of healthy fats in the diet, as these essential fatty acids are needed for an efficient metabolism.

  Conversely, it is wise to avoid the unhealthy fats, which can lead to a fatty liver.

While trying to lose weight, the fats to avoid are:

1. deep-fried foods
2. hydrogenated vegetable oils (read the labels)
3. full-cream dairy products – cream, ice-cream and butter
4. margarines containing transfatty acids and hydrogenated oils
5. the fats found in preserved meats.

While trying to lose weight, get your healthy fats from foods such as:

1. seafood – all types are suitable
2. eggs – preferably organic
3. fresh lean red and white meat
4. tahini, hummus, nut spreads
5. avocado
6. raw nuts and seeds
7. cold-pressed seed and vegetable oils.

Don't be fooled by promoters of the 'low-fat' approach to weight loss. If you follow a very low-fat, low-calorie diet, your metabolism will slow down, so that when you stop the diet you will put on weight more rapidly than before. You could become a yo-yo dieter. Fat does not raise insulin levels, so for those with Syndrome X, fat is not the primary enemy, provided your fats are chosen from healthy sources.

Many dieticians now realize that patients with Syndrome X do not respond well in the long term to low-fat, low-calorie, high-carbohydrate diets.

The reasons that my Syndrome X programme is so successful for weight loss is that it lowers insulin levels, which achieves several benefits:

1. It reduces your appetite, especially for carbohydrates.
2. It reduces cravings for sugar.
3. It increases energy levels and the ability to exercise.

4. It reduces the storage of body fat.
5. It increases the body's ability to burn its fat stores for energy.

At our weight loss clinic in Sydney we see many very overweight people who weigh above 140 kg (22 stone). These people have usually tried everything, and they really need a programme that is going to curb their appetite. They usually tell me how relieved they are to be able to eat when they feel hungry, and not to have to go on a starvation diet. For victims of Syndrome X, the most important thing is what they eat, not *how much* they eat. Weight loss is gradual, with an average loss of 1 to 2 kg (2 to 4 pounds) a week; however, the weight loss is permanent if they stick to the golden rules as found on pages 115–18. They eventually lose an enormous amount of weight once we get their liver working efficiently and their insulin levels down.

## HEALTHY MENUS FOR WEIGHT LOSS

Breakfast Ideas

2 to 3 boiled eggs with a salad of fruits and raw vegetables

Egg and mixed-vegetable omelette

Muesli with *no* added sugar

Smoothie – Protein powder, lite coconut milk or skimmed milk, soymilk or oat milk, water and fresh fruits in season. Fresh berries of all varieties are excellent for weight loss.

Fresh fruit salad with cottage or ricotta cheese

Grilled fish or sardines with salad

Stoneground wholemeal bread with cottage cheese and salad or seasonal fruits

Rolled oats with skimmed milk – add some raw nuts and seeds to make this a complete protein meal

If you start the day with first-class proteins instead of carbohydrates alone, your insulin levels will remain lower during the day.

This is desirable for those with a weight problem, as high insulin levels turn carbohydrate into body fat, and they also stimulate hunger and cravings for more carbohydrates. This is very important if you are going to lose weight successfully, and I am often surprised by the number of women who do not eat adequate protein regularly. No wonder they have a weight problem, as their metabolism has been trained to store fat. In those who are metabolically resistant, you will need to avoid breakfasts containing any cereals or grains until you have achieved a satisfactory weight loss first.

Lunch and Dinner Ideas

Grilled fish with vegetables and salad
Grilled chicken with vegetables and salad
Salad with avocado and mixed beans, nuts and seeds
Egg salad or omelette
Lamb and vegetable soup or stew, and salad
Fish, lamb or beef curry with brown rice/lentils and vegetables
Tofu curry with brown rice/lentils and vegetables – sprinkle
    with sesame seeds
Stir-fried vegetables with chicken, meat or seafood

If you are metabolically resistant avoid the rice and replace it
    with lentils, chickpeas or soy beans.

High Protein Snack Ideas

**Protein Smoothie**

Place in a blender –

1 cup coconut milk diluted 50 per cent with water, or lite coconut
    milk, or soy milk (no added sugar)
2 scoops Protein Powder (for details of where to get the brand
    Synd-X, visit www.weightcontroldoctor.com)
Fresh berries of choice – raspberries, blackberries, blueberries,
    gooseberries, strawberries
Ice if desired

This smoothie tastes sweet, because the Synd-X Protein Powder is sweetened with the naturally sweet herb called stevia, and natural vanilla flavour. Stevia is calorie free. Synd-X Slimming Protein Powder also contains added chromium picolinate, taurine and glutamine.

This is a delicious creamy smoothie that is low in carbohydrate. The natural fruit acids in the berries have the ability to lower insulin levels.

**Vegetarian 'On the Run' First-Class Protein Snack Pack**
Roasted legumes – beans and chickpeas
Almonds
Brazil nuts
Sunflower seeds
Dried apricot
Dried apple
Flaked coconut

This snack-pack tastes delicious and is very filling, so that you don't feel like snacking for hours. Indeed, it tastes much better than packaged snacks such as crisps or pretzels, which are loaded with carbohydrate and hydrogenated oils and will send your insulin levels soaring. You can make this Snack Pack yourself, as you can find the ingredients in most health food shops. This snack provides first-class protein, as it combines legumes, nuts and seeds together. It's also high in fibre, which benefits those with sluggish bowels and constipation.

Many sufferers of Syndrome X experience strong and unpredictable cravings for carbohydrates, and they need to be prepared with protein snacks to fight back. Yes, it can be difficult trying to lose weight if you are not prepared for the battle of the cravings.

You can keep protein snacks handy so that they are immediately available, when you are attacked by a craving.

### Other Good Protein Snacks

1. Small tins of tuna, salmon or real crab meat
2. Sealed container of fresh vegetable salad with chopped hard boiled eggs or feta, parmesan or cottage cheese. Dressing of cold-pressed oil, lemon or apple cider vinegar.
3. Fresh fruit with ricotta or cottage cheese

If you enjoy tea and coffee, you may sweeten these beverages with the naturally sweet herb called stevia. You can also add stevia to desserts, sauces and home-made lemonade.

Stevia is calorie free and does not raise blood sugar levels, and thus is an ideal sweetener for weight watchers. Stevia has been studied extensively and has been found to be non-toxic and safe to use by people with diabetes. Stevia is available in tablets or white powder, and only tiny amounts need to be used, as stevia is 300 times sweeter than sugar. The availability of stevia means that it is now easy to avoid artificial sweeteners.

## Natural Supplements to Help Insulin Work Better

Studies have shown that there are specific herbs, antioxidants, vitamins and minerals that can improve the function of insulin. This is most beneficial because, if we can reduce insulin resistance, the pancreas will not have to produce such high levels of insulin. With lower levels of insulin, the process of fat-burning can begin!

Studies have shown that the minerals *magnesium* and *chromium* can improve the function of insulin. Chromium picolinate is a well absorbed and effective form of chromium.

*Lipoic acid* is an antioxidant that has been shown to improve glucose metabolism and is recommended to reduce the complications of diabetes.

*Carnitine* is a protein that helps the conversion of food energy into cellular energy and improves metabolism.

The herbs *Momordica Charantia (Bitter Melon)* and *Gymnema Sylvestre* can exert a favourable effect upon carbohydrate metabolism.

The amino acids *glutamine* and *taurine* help the function of insulin and also the liver, which aids weight loss.

Many people who are plagued with sugar cravings find that these herbs and nutrients greatly reduce their cravings. They can be taken individually, or are available combined together in supplement form.

For more information visit www.weightcontroldoctor.com

## DETOXIFICATION AND WEIGHT LOSS

If you are overweight and feel generally tired and sluggish, and yet all your tests come back normal, you may find yourself reju-venated by a gentle two-day detoxification programme. The best time to do this is when you do not have to work, so a weekend or holiday period is probably best. I recommend a two-day raw juice and vegetable soup fast, to cleanse the liver, bowel and lymphatic system. You will need a juicer.

**Morning Juice** (on rising)

1 apple

2 carrots

3 sticks celery

¼ bunch parsley (optional)

**Lunchtime Juice**

2 leaves cabbage

5 green beans

2 spinach leaves or 2 fresh dandelion leaves

2 red apples

**Afternoon Juice**

1 orange

1 grapefruit or lime

1 kiwi fruit

1-cm slice fresh ginger root

1 carrot

1 cucumber (with its skin)

**Dinnertime Soup for 2 nights**

| | |
|---|---|
| 1 tbsp | cold-pressed olive oil |
| 2 | potatoes, chopped |
| 1 | carrot, chopped |
| 1 | onion, chopped |
| 2 cloves | garlic, peeled and crushed (optional) |
| 32 fl oz | water |
| 1 bunch | spinach, washed and shredded |
| 6 oz / 180 g | green beans |
| 1 floret | broccoli |
| 4 oz / 120 g | chopped parsley |
| 2 tbsps | miso paste |
| | salt and pepper to taste |

**place** oil into a large saucepan on medium heat

**add** potatoes, carrot, onion and garlic and stir until the onion is soft

**pour** in the water

**bring** to the boil and turn down to a simmer

**when** potatoes are nearly cooked, add the other vegetables

**when** they are cooked, turn off the heat

**add** the miso and stir through until dissolved

When reheating the soup for the next evening, do not boil (as it destroys the enzymes in the miso), but bring to a simmer until heated through.

**Evening Beverage**

Herbal teas – red clover, peppermint, sage or chamomile – sweetened with stevia, if desired

Make sure that you drink 10 glasses of water during the day, in between juices.

This gentle detox will improve liver function and enable increased elimination of toxins through the bowels and urine. You will find that this helps you to control your weight and greatly improves the complexion. Most people find that they have increased energy levels for at least one week after this detox.

If you get excellent results, you may repeat this two-day cleansing on a regular basis. Although organic juices are ideal, you will still achieve great benefit if you choose any fresh produce that is in season.

### Case History

Maggie was typical of many women who come to see me trying to restore balance in their lives. For many women, physical and emotional balance can be elusive, especially since we cannot achieve one without the other. Maggie was 44 years old and had gained 27 kg (4 stone 3) since going through the menopause two years before. She was an apple-shaped woman, carrying all her excessive weight in the abdominal area, and had a roll of fat around her upper abdomen.

She forced herself to avoid eating, but even when she did this she did not lose weight. Her doctor had given her high doses of the hormone oestrogen in tablet form. Maggie did not realize that she had a fatty liver, and her poor, dysfunctional liver could not cope with the strong hormones she was taking. Understandably they had caused more weight gain, and Maggie was trapped in a vicious circle of ever-increasing weight.

After testing Maggie I confirmed that she had a fatty liver and slightly high cholesterol, triglyceride and insulin levels. She also felt hungry most of the time. Maggie was relieved to discover that she had a specific diagnosis of fatty liver and Syndrome X, to explain why she could not lose weight.

I stopped her oestrogen tablets and gave her a hormone cream containing natural Triest (see page 74) and progesterone.

This cream would be much better for her overworked liver, which could now get on with its job of burning fat.

Maggie loved protein and vegetables, so the Syndrome X eating plan was easy for her to follow. She found that her hunger was easily controlled by avoiding carbohydrates such as breads, biscuits, crackers, chips, noodles, rice and pasta. She had thought these things were helping her, but in Syndrome X these high-carbohydrate foods only increase the appetite. I also gave Maggie a supplement to reduce the chemical imbalance caused by Syndrome X.

Over a six-month period Maggie lost 23 kg (3½ stone) and also lost her potbelly. She had found this weight-loss process to be effective and easy, as the eating plan had lowered her insulin levels, which had reduced her appetite. Insulin is not only a fat-storing hormone, it also increases the appetite.

Maggie was now able to fit into her old clothes and wear attractive belts again.

I have found that many women with a dysfunctional or a fatty liver are taking inappropriate Hormone Replacement Therapy (HRT) which aggravates their obesity. In such cases it is not wise to take tablets containing strong or synthetic hormones, as these will increase the workload of the liver. I recommend hormone creams or patches containing natural oestrogen and progesterone, as these are absorbed directly through the skin and bypass the liver. If we can reduce the workload of the liver, it will be more efficient at burning fat.

### Case History

Ruth, aged 49, suffered from type 2 diabetes, controlled with diet and medication; she had started to experience palpitations, hot flushes and disturbed sleep over the previous two months. Her weight continued to increase, and she had gone from 68 kg (10 stone 10) to 79 kg (12 stone 5) over the previous six months. Ruth had a large appetite and craved carbohydrates such as bread and sweets, although she knew they made her feel very tired. She had found it impossible to lose weight. She wanted to take something natural for her menopause, as she had read that women with diabetes cannot take HRT.

When I examined Ruth, I found that her blood pressure was mildly elevated and her heart beat was irregular. I referred her to a cardiologist for further tests.

She returned to see me four weeks later, and thankfully the cardiologist had not found any underlying problem with her heart. He had told her that her problems were related to her excess weight and diabetes, and recommended that she try and lose weight quickly.

Blood tests revealed that Ruth had very low levels of oestradiol, and high levels of FSH (see page 37), thus confirming that she was now truly menopausal. She had all the biochemical abnormalities of Syndrome X – elevated triglyceride fats, high LDL cholesterol, and elevated fasting insulin levels.

I explained to Ruth that we could overcome the majority of her problems if we could reduce her insulin levels back to normal. Her high levels of insulin were causing her body to store fat and preventing her from burning fat. Her high insulin levels were making her crave carbohydrates, which after eating, further elevated her insulin levels. So poor Ruth felt trapped in a metabolic nightmare, and the harder she tried to lose weight, the less success she had.

The first step to help her was to get her to follow an eating plan. Just to give you a brief outline of the changes she had to make in her diet for the first 12 weeks, I have designed a little chart. This helps you to see at a glance how easy these changes are.

| RUTH'S NORMAL DIET | RUTH'S WEIGHT LOSS DIET |
|---|---|
| **Breakfast** | **Breakfast** |
| Wholegrain bread, margarine, packaged cereal, milk, black coffee with artificial sweetener | Fresh vegetable juice – one glass 2 to 3 eggs – poached, boiled or scrambled, or as an omelette with added chopped vegetables One piece fruit (apple or citrus or kiwi fruit) **Or** Synd-X Protein Powder Smoothie – lite coconut milk, fresh berries, 2 scoops protein powder If desired, coffee with stevia to sweeten |
| **Lunch** | **Lunch** |
| Sandwich – cheese, ham, small amount salad **Or** Pasta with creamy sauce **Or** Chinese takeaway Coffee with artificial sweetener | Bowl fresh salad with fresh chicken, prawns, tuna, salmon, or a combination of cooked beans, toasted sesame seeds and raw almonds **Or** Cheese (parmesan, feta, ricotta or cottage) with a large bowl of salad, a few nuts and seeds added **Or** Cheese (parmesan, feta, ricotta or cottage) with 2 fresh fruit pieces, a few raw nuts and seeds added Dressing of cold-pressed oil & lemon, or apple cider vinegar on all salads, if desired |
| **Dinner** | **Dinner** |
| Pasta with creamy sauce and vegetables **Or** Stir-fry vegetables, meat & rice **Or** | Stir-fry meat, chicken, or seafood with vegetables (no rice) **Or** Steak or grilled fish and vegetables **Or** |

| | |
|---|---|
| Vegetable and chicken soup with large amounts of crusty bread<br>Low-fat flavoured yogurt<br>Biscuits and cheese | Chicken and vegetable soup<br>Lamb and vegetable casserole<br>Salad to be served with all meals – dressing of cold pressed oil and lemon, or apple cider vinegar<br>2 tbsp plain yogurt with 1 piece of real fruit |
| **Snacks**<br>Biscuits and cheese and ham<br>Low-fat cookies<br>Crisps and low-fat pretzels<br>Bread and Marmite<br>Bread and ham<br>Diabetic chocolate and jams (artificially sweetened)<br>Diet sodas | **Snacks**<br>Cheese – parmesan, ricotta, cottage or feta, with sticks of celery and carrot, or 1 piece of fresh fruit<br>Raw nuts<br>Synd-X High Protein Snack Pack<br>Small can of seafood (tuna, salmon, sardines or crab meat)<br>Smoothie made with High Protein Powder with fresh berries.<br>Cheese – parmesan, ricotta or feta with raw nuts |

Ruth found it easy to adapt to this eating plan, as because it was low in carbohydrate it did not stimulate her insulin levels to become higher. Because insulin makes you feel hungry, especially for carbohydrates, Ruth found that on this eating plan her appetite was much reduced. Over a period of four months she lost 10 kg (1½ stone) and was down to 69 kg (10 stone 12). Her blood sugar levels came down, so that I was gradually able to take her off her diabetes medication. Her blood pressure came down and her palpitations ceased and she felt much calmer, as she was no longer plagued by unstable blood sugar levels. I repeated her glucose tolerance test, and this came back within normal levels, so that Ruth was no longer technically suffering from diabetes.

Ruth was still keen to get some treatment for her menopausal symptoms, as she was troubled by hot flushes, sweating and vaginal dryness. I prescribed a cream containing natural oestrogen combined with natural progesterone. Ruth was told to massage this cream into the skin of her inner upper thigh, every night on retiring.

For women prone to weight gain and diabetes, I prefer to use creams containing only natural hormones, as they do not place any strain upon the liver. Conversely, oral hormones, especially the synthetic progestogens, could possibly aggravate poor blood sugar control and high cholesterol levels.

## Recipes High in Phytoestrogens and Protein

### bean niçoise serves 4

| | |
|---|---|
| 225g / 8 oz | cherry tomatoes |
| 1½ tbsp | cold pressed olive oil |
| 2 tbsp | fresh chives, chopped |
| 225g / 8 oz | snap beans, chopped into 2-cm lengths |
| 4 | small eggs, boiled, peeled and cut in half |
| 1 tin | butter beans, rinsed |
| 1 tin | borlotti beans, rinsed |
| 140g / 5 oz | fresh peas |
| 1 | red onion, thinly sliced |
| 100g / 3½ oz | small black olives |
| 60g / 2 oz cup | walnuts or 2 tbsp toasted sesame seeds |
| | sea salt and pepper to taste |

dressing

| | |
|---|---|
| 1 | egg |
| 2 | anchovy fillets |
| 1 | clove garlic, crushed |
| 1 | lime, juiced |
| 1 tsp | Dijon mustard |
| ½ tsp | Worcestershire sauce (tamari can be used instead) |
| 160ml / 5fl oz | cold-pressed olive oil |

| place | all the dressing ingredients into a food processor |
|---|---|
| blend | and set aside |
| cut | tomatoes in half and season |
| toss | in half the chives and ½ tsp olive oil, mix |
| place | tomatoes cut side down on a tray in the oven |
| bake | for 20 min until slightly wilted |
| bring | pan of water to boil |
| add | round beans and cook for 1 min |
| drain | and run under cold water |
| mix | peas, borlotti and butter beans together in a bowl |
| place | a portion of bean mix in each serving bowl |
| add | a few slivers of onion to each dish |
| add | the round beans |
| place | in each bowl the egg, olives and tomatoes |
| drizzle | the dressing over each bowl |
| serve | with the remaining chives, walnuts or sesame seeds sprinkled on top |

## eggs in a spicy tomato sauce serves 2

Great for breakfast, lunch or dinner

| | |
|---|---|
| 4 | large free-range eggs |
| 2 tbsp | olive oil |
| 1 | onion, peeled and chopped |
| 1 tsp | ground cumin seeds |
| 1 tsp | ground coriander |
| 1 | red chilli, diced |
| 3 | cloves garlic, peeled and crushed |
| 2 | red capsicum, deseeded and diced finely |
| 1 tin | tomatoes, drained and chopped – keep the juice to the side |
| 2 | bunches spinach, washed sea salt and fresh black pepper to taste |

| place | spinach in a large saucepan, over medium heat |
|---|---|
| **add** | salt and pepper to taste |
| **cover** | the spinach with a lid and steam until wilted |
| **stirfry** | onions until slightly brown in a large frying pan on medium heat |
| **add** | garlic, chilli, cumin seeds and diced capsicum |
| **stir in** | coriander until the peppers begin to soften |
| **add** | tomatoes and salt and pepper to taste |
| | when the sauce is simmering, make four spaces for the eggs |
| **crack** | the eggs into the spaces provided and lower the heat |
| **cover** | the pan, cook gently for a few minutes until eggs are done to your liking |
| **divide** | the spinach |
| **add** | eggs and sauce serve immediately |

## chickpea and pumpkin cakes serves 4

| | |
|---|---|
| 1 tin | chickpeas, drained and rinsed |
| 1 | red onion, finely chopped |
| 2 tbsp | chickpea flour |
| 315g / 11 oz | pumpkin, peeled, seeded and chopped |
| 2 tbsp | flat leafed parsley, chopped |
| 60ml / 2 fl oz | cold-pressed olive oil |
| | sea salt and pepper to taste |

| | |
|---|---|
| **cook** | pumpkin in boiling water until soft |
| **drain** | and transfer into a large bowl |
| **add** | half the chickpeas and mash until smooth |
| **toss in** | onion, flour, remaining chickpeas and parsley |
| **add** | salt and pepper to taste |
| **mix** | thoroughly and make into approx 16 patties |
| **heat** | olive oil in a large frying pan |
| **add** | patties and cook 2–3 min each side |

**serve**     immediately with the **tomato, alfalfa and**
          **cucumber salad** (see page 139)
Swede can be used in place of pumpkin.

## broadbeans, asparagus and miso serves 4

| | |
|---|---|
| 455g / 16 oz | shelled broadbeans |
| 240ml / 8 fl oz | vegetable stock |
| 1½ tsp | tamari |
| 1 tbsp | miso paste |
| 1 tbsp | shredded ginger |
| 3 | bunches green asparagus, trimmed and halved |
| 115g / 4 oz | mangetout, trimmed |
| 140g / 5 oz | oyster mushrooms (button can be used also) |
| 2 tsp | sesame seeds |
| 60g / 2 oz | nuts of choice (pecan, walnuts, cashews) |
| 1 tsp | cold pressed olive oil |

**place**     broadbeans in a pan of simmering water
**cook**     for 2 min, drain, cool and peel
**mix**     miso, stock and tamari, set aside
**heat**     wok (frying pan) on high with oil
**add**     ginger and cook for 1 min
**add**     asparagus cook for a further 2 min
**add**     snow peas, mushrooms and miso mixture
**stirfry**     until asparagus is tender (approx 2 min)
**stir in**     broadbeans until warmed
**serve**     sprinkled with sesame seeds and nuts

## walnut and bean salad serves 2
This dish can be served on its own, or also as a side dish with
any vegetable, meat, fish, tofu or tempeh dish

| | |
|---|---|
| ¹⁄₂ | Cos or iceburg lettuce, rinsed and torn into bite-size pieces |
| ¹⁄₂ | red cabbage, rinsed and sliced into thin shreds |
| ¹⁄₂ bunch | spinach, washed and roughly chopped |
| 1 | avocado, peeled and chopped into bite-size chunks |
| 2 | med ripe tomatoes chopped into bite size chunks |
| 1 | med beet, peeled and grated |
| 2 | stalks of celery, washed and chopped into slithers |
| 140g / 5 oz | fresh peas |
| 115g / 4 oz | steamed snap beans |
| 2 | spring onions, thinly sliced into rounds |
| 170g / 6 oz | cooked chick peas |
| 1 tbsp | toasted sunflower seeds |
| 2 tbsp | walnuts roughly crushed |
| 1 handful | alfalfa sprouts |
| | |
| **toss** | all together in a large bowl |
| **serve** | with your favourite dressing |

## stuffed tomatoes serves 4

This stuffing is great for many vegetables

| | |
|---|---|
| 8 | medium, firm, ripe tomatoes |

**stuffing mixture**

| | |
|---|---|
| 3 | free-range eggs |
| 10 | basil leaves, rinsed and chopped |
| 1 | clove of garlic, peeled and finely chopped or crushed |
| 5 tbsp | cooked green or red lentils |
| 3 tbsp | freshly grated parmesan |
| 1 tbsp | lemon juice |
| 2 tbsp | parsley, rinsed and chopped |
| | sea salt and freshly ground black pepper to taste |

**break**   eggs into a bowl and lightly beat

| | |
|---|---|
| **add** | remaining ingredients and stir well |

**to assemble the tomatoes**

| | |
|---|---|
| **heat** | oven to 200°C / 400°F / GM 6 |
| **cut** | tomatoes in half and scoop out the seeds |
| **turn** | the tomatoes upside down and let them drain for 20 minutes |
| **place** | tomatoes in a baking dish |
| **divide** | stuffing between them |
| **bake** | in the oven for 15 minutes until the tomatoes are tender (you don't want them to lose their shape) |
| **let cool** | for 5 minutes before serving; can also be served at room temperature |

## eastern omelette serves 2

| | |
|---|---|
| 3 tbsp | cold-pressed olive oil |
| 1 | carrot, grated |
| 115g / 4 oz | Chinese cabbage, shredded |
| 170g / 6 oz | beansprouts |
| 6 | spring onions sliced diagonally (thinly) |
| 8 | mushrooms, wiped and sliced thinly |
| 115g / 4 oz | mangetout, trimmed and sliced in three |
| 1 | small red chilli, finely chopped (optional) |
| 2 tsp | tamari or light soy |
| 2 tsp | toasted sesame seed oil |
| 60g / 2 oz | cilantro leaves, washed |
| 4 | large free-range eggs |
| | sea salt and pepper to taste |

| | |
|---|---|
| **heat** | wok until hot |
| **add** | 1 tbsp of olive oil |
| **toss in** | vegetables, chilli and stir-fry over high heat for 2 min |
| **add** | tamari, sesame oil and coriander |

| **stirfry** | for 30 seconds |
| **whisk** | 2 eggs with 1tbsp water and season to taste |
| **heat** | 2 tbsp olive oil in a 24cm non-stick frying pan |
| **add** | egg mixture and cook on high heat |
| **swivel** | the pan so that the egg mixture runs to the edges |
| **cook** | for 2–3 min until almost set |
| **place** | half the vegetable mixture on one side of the omelette |
| **fold** | over the omelette onto the vegetable mixture |
| **remove** | from pan onto a warm plate |
| **repeat** | process for the other omelette |
| **serve** | drizzled with tamari |

## chickpea salad with haloumi serves 2–4

Haloumi is a white, salty cheese from Cyprus. Cook and serve immediately; if you leave the cheese too long it will become rubbery.

| 2 tins | chickpeas, rinsed and drained |
| 1 tbsp | lemon juice |
| 2 tbsp | parsley, chopped |
| 2 tbsp | coriander, chopped |
| 4 tbsp | olive oil |
| 1 | garlic clove, peeled and crushed |
| 1 | dash tamari |
| 1 | chilli, diced (optional although very tasty) |
| ½ | small red onion finely diced |
| 230g /8 oz | haloumi |
| 100g / 3½ oz | rocket, rinsed (or baby spinach) |
| 100g / 3½ oz | black olives |
| 12 | medium ripe tomatoes |
| | sea salt and pepper to taste |

| **heat** | oven to 200°C / 400°F / GM 6 |
| **cut** | tomatoes in half and place on an oiled baking tray |
| **drizzle** | 2 tbsp of oil over the tomatoes, roast in oven |

until they look chewy

**mix** chickpeas, lemon juice, fresh herbs, remaining oil,
garlic, in a large bowl

**add** chilli, onion, tamari, salt and pepper to taste
and mix well

**cut** haloumi into 2-cm thick slices, rinse and pat dry
baste the haloumi with olive oil

**divide** enough chickpea mixture into bowls for serving

**add** roasted tomatoes and black olives

**place** small non-stick frying pan on high heat

**cook** the haloumi approx 1 minute each side until
golden brown

**place** cheese quickly on top of salad and serve immediately

## mixed vegetable dinner serves 2–4

This is a quick, easy and delicious meal. Great to take to work,
cold the next day. Don't worry about trying to keep everything
warm – it's fine to have some things at room temperature or cold.

### tempeh chips

Great to have with steamed vegetables or salads, or when you
need a boost of protein

315g / 11 oz     tempeh cut into little finger-size lengths
3 tbsp           olive oil
splash           tamari (optional)

**put** 3 tbsp of oil into a wok or large frying pan

**turn** the heat to high

**toss in** the tempeh and stir-fry until golden brown
(about 5 minutes)

**stir in** the tamari (optional)
remove and place to the side

### ginger spinach

| | |
|---|---|
| 2 bunches | spinach, washed |
| 1 tbsp | olive oil |
| 1 tbsp | fresh ginger, peeled and sliced into the size of matches |
| 2 tbsp | sesame seeds |
| 1 splash | tamari (optional) |
| | sea salt and pepper to taste |

**place** oil into a large saucepan over high heat
**add** ginger, pepper and salt to taste, then the sesame seeds
**stir** for 2 minutes
**toss in** the spinach, use pepper and salt throughout the spinach
**stirfry** until wilted (about 5 minutes)

### mushrooms

| | |
|---|---|
| 230g / 8oz | mushrooms |
| 2 tbsp | olive oil |
| | sea salt and pepper to taste |

**place** all ingredients into a saucepan on a high heat
**cook** until mushrooms are tender

### swede

| | |
|---|---|
| 570g / 20 oz | swede (skin removed), cut into bite-size pieces |
| 1 splash | tamari |
| 1 | clove garlic, diced very finely |
| | sea salt and pepper to taste |

**place** all ingredients into a baking tray and stir
**bake** until cooked

## lentils

| | |
|---|---|
| 600g / 21 oz | cooked lentils (green or brown) |
| 1 | onion, peeled and sliced |
| 1 | clove garlic, crushed |
| 2 tbsp | cold pressed olive oil (optional) |
| | sea salt and pepper to taste |

**stirfry** onions and garlic in a non-stick frying pan
**add** lentils and salt and pepper
**stir** until warmed through

## tomato, alfalfa and cucumber salad

| | |
|---|---|
| 455g / 16 oz | firm tomatoes, chopped |
| 2 | lebanese cucumbers, chopped |
| 90g / 3 oz | alfalfa sprouts |
| 2 tbsp | cold-pressed flax seed or olive oil |
| 1 | red onion, diced finely |
| 1/2 | lettuce, washed and torn into small pieces |

place all ingredients into a bowl and mix through

## chickpea soup serves 6

| | |
|---|---|
| 5 tbsp | cold-pressed olive oil |
| 1 | med onion, roughly chopped |
| 200g / 7 oz | brown lentils |
| 230g / 8 oz | broadbeans, soaked over night |
| 170g / 6 oz | chickpeas, soaked over night |
| 690g / 24 oz | tomatoes, roughly chopped |
| 1 | whole celery head, including green leaf, chopped |
| 1 | vegetable (dark in colour) stock cube |
| 2 | cloves garlic, finely sliced |
| 2 tsp | cumin powder |
| 2 1/4 l / 3 1/2 pt | water |
| 2 tbsp | chickpea flour |

| | |
|---|---|
| 1 | lemon, juiced |
| 1 pinch | cayenne pepper |
| 1 bunch | parsley, finely chopped |
| 1 bunch | cilantro, finely chopped |
| 1 red chilli | (optional), finely diced |
| | sea salt and pepper to taste |

**heat** oil in a large saucepan

**add** onion and cook until transparent

**add** crumbled stock cube, celery, chilli and lentils and

**cook** stirring for 3 minutes

**toss in** chickpeas, broadbeans, tomatoes, cumin, some black pepper and garlic and stir through

**pour** in the water

**cover** with a lid and simmer for approx one hour or until the beans are tender

**place** the flour in a small bowl and some of the hot liquid from the soup and make a paste

**return** the paste to soup and stir through until it thickens

**add** the lemon juice, parsley, coriander and seasoning to taste

**remove** from heat and stir

**serve** with a big green salad

## alfalfa salad serves 1–3

| | |
|---|---|
| 1 | punnet fresh alfalfa sprouts |
| 1 | head lettuce, washed and shredded |
| 6 | red radishes, washed and sliced thinly |
| 1 | lebanese cucumber, sliced into thin rounds |
| 1 | carrot, washed and grated |
| 1 | beet, peeled and grated |
| 140g / 5 oz | fresh peas |
| 1 tin | borlotti beans, drained and rinsed |
| 170g / 6 oz | fresh corn kernels, removed from cob |

| 60g / 2 oz | slivered almonds |
| dressing | |
| 2 tbsp | toasted sesame seeds |
| 1 | lemon, juiced |
| 2 tbsp | cold-pressed olive oil |
| 1 tsp | seeded mustard |

**place** all ingredients for the salad in a large bowl and toss

**place** all ingredients for the dressing into a jar and shake

**pour** the dressing over the salad and serve

## aduki bean rolls serves 1–3

| 200g / 7 oz | aduki beans, soaked overnight, then cooked till soft |
| 2 | cloves garlic, crushed and marinated in oil |
| 2 tbsp | cold-pressed olive oil for the garlic |
| 140g / 5 oz | tahini |
| 1 tbsp | flaxseeds, ground |
| 1 tsp | cumin powder |
| 3 tbsp | lemon juice |
| 30g / 1 oz | parsley, chopped |
| 115g / 4 oz | onion, diced |
| 230g / 8 oz | sesame seeds toasted |

**drain** and mash the beans

**heat** a wok on medium heat and add the garlic and oil mix

**remove** the garlic and add the onions and simmer til soft

**blend** ½ cup of the mashed beans with the onion and garlic

**add** the remaining beans, tahini, flaxseeds, cumin, lemon juice and parsley, and blend

**set** aside the mixture to cool

**shape** into 2 logs and roll in the sesame seeds

**serve** with a vegetable salad

# Chapter 9

# Body Types and HRT

Have you ever wondered 'What does my body type have to do with the type of hormone replacement that is best for me?'

Good question, because it has practical implications. I have observed over many years that there are basically four different body types (or shapes), and each type has interesting hormonal and metabolic differences. These differences make it easy to understand why different women, need different types of HRT. Anyway, understanding your Body Type is fun!

I know this, because when I do seminars everyone in the audience lines up in a queue until they are examined and told what body type they are. Sometimes they wait for hours, just to find this out.

*To know your Body Type NOW you need to do an interactive questionnaire – to do this visit* www.weightcontroldoctor.com. Each of the four body types may be short, medium or tall in height.

To help you understand how your body type may affect the type of HRT that is best for you, I have designed a little table to make it easy. Of course this is a generalization, but you will be amazed just how often this works out to be true!

I love tables because they make things easy – you can pick the part that interests you, and see the information at a glance.

| YOUR BODY TYPE | DESCRIPTION OF BODY SHAPE | HORMONAL CHARACTERISTICS | BEST TYPE OF HRT |
|---|---|---|---|
| **ANDROID** | Broad shoulders and narrow hips. Does not go in at the waist. Strong muscular shapely legs and arms. Puts on weight in the upper part of the body and abdomen. Can become apple shaped. | May suffer with Syndrome X (insulin excess). May have a sluggish liver, or a fatty liver. May overproduce male hormones from the fat tissue in the upper body, especially if she is overweight. Often low in progesterone. | Transdermal – eg. patches, creams, or gels containing natural oestrogen and progesterone. Rarely needs testosterone. |
| **GYNAEOID** | Medium shoulders, narrow waist and very curvy. Wide hips. Fine ankles and wrists. The weight goes on the buttocks, hips and thighs so that a pear shape may result. | More likely to suffer with 'oestrogen dominance' and a relative deficiency of progesterone. This may result in PMS, heavy painful periods or endometriosis. Many women, especially Gynaeoid types, continue to make plenty of oestrone in the fat of the lower body, even years after the menopause. | May need to take only progesterone in the form of a cream, lozenge or micronised capsule. If oestrogen is used, use only a small dose, as excess oestrogen will cause fat to increase on the buttocks, hips and thighs. Weaker oestrogens such as oestriol can be more suitable. |

| YOUR BODY TYPE | DESCRIPTION OF BODY SHAPE | HORMONAL CHARACTERISTICS | BEST TYPE OF HRT |
|---|---|---|---|
| **LYMPHATIC** | The excess weight is deposited all over the body. They tend to put on weight very easily, due to a very low metabolic rate. There is fluid retention because the lymphatic system is dysfunctional. The limbs are thick and puffy. The bone structure is not very evident. | Because weight gain occurs all over the body, many types of hormonal imbalances may arise. They are prone to Syndrome X and thyroid underactivity. Lymphatics are also prone to oestrogen dominance, and progesterone deficiency. Often we find that their levels of male hormones are naturally adequate, or even too high, especially if they have Syndrome X. | Because they are prone to fluid retention, they should avoid oral forms of hormones. Transdermal hormones are best, such as patches, creams or gels. It is best to us the weaker oestrogens, such as oestriol or oestrone. Sometimes all that is needed is natural progesterone. |

| YOUR BODY TYPE | DESCRIPTION OF BODY SHAPE | HORMONAL CHARACTERISTICS | BEST TYPE OF HRT |
|---|---|---|---|
| **THYROID** | Fine bone structure. They have long limbs, compared to the trunk, which makes them look taller than they are. They are often slim or thin. Do not put on weight easily, as they have a high metabolic rate and often crave stimulants. | Thyroid types may have a later puberty, and/or an earlier menopause. The size of their endocrine glands may be smaller, and this, combined with their low body fat, means that they often produce lower amounts of sex hormones and other steroid hormones. This makes them more likely to suffer with adrenal gland exhaustion and osteoporosis. | They may have severe menopausal symptoms because their level of hormone deficiency is often much greater, especially if they are underweight and/or smoke. Thus we often need to use higher doses of natural hormones. We also often need to give a greater range of hormones, such as DHEA, testosterone, oestrogen and progesterone. |

# Chapter 10

# The Menopause and Your Appearance

## What Can I Do about Hair Loss?

As we age our hair often deteriorates and we need to spend more time looking after it.

The biggest problem for women is hair loss during the menopause, and this is a frequent problem we get asked about at the Health Advisory Service. Most women find hair loss very distressing, and many have difficulty getting help.

Hair loss is common during the peri-menopausal years, partly because of the gradual decline of the female sex hormones oestrogen and progesterone. This can cause the hair to become finer and more dull. Many women find that their hair improves on natural hormone replacement therapy, and becomes less dry. Natural progesterone is particularly good for the hair, and usually thickens it up.

Some women produce excessive male hormones; this is a common cause of hair loss. We find this especially in women with the following problems:

### POLYCYSTIC OVARIAN SYNDROME (PCOS)

In these women ovulation does not occur regularly, so there is a resultant lack of progesterone. Their male hormones may be very high, as determined with the measurement of the Free Androgen Index (FAI) by blood test. The free androgens are the male hormones that circulate in the bloodstream unbound to proteins, and because they are unbound, they are very active. These male hormones cause thinning of the hair in the male pattern – namely on the top and sides of the scalp.

## OVERWEIGHT

Excessive male hormones are also often found in women who are overweight with most of the weight being carried in the upper part of the body and the abdomen. These women gain weight in the trunk, the arms and the abdominal area. Upper-level body fat produces male hormones which can reach very high levels, as determined by the measurement of the Free Androgen Index. Weight loss reduces the amount of male hormones, with a resultant reduction in hair loss.

Natural progesterone can help women with male hormone-induced hair loss. If the male hormones are very high, it may be necessary to prescribe an anti-male hormone called cyproterone acetate, which blocks the effects of the male hormones upon the skin and hair follicles. Cyproterone can greatly reduce male hormone-induced hair loss, as well as excess facial and body hair. The drug called aldosterone is sometimes prescribed for hair loss, but it is not as effective as cyproterone acetate.

Cyproterone can be prescribed with a small dose of natural oestrogen, to make the hormonal profile more feminine, which will thicken the hair. When we reduce the excessive male hormones, weight loss is often easier, as male hormones increase insulin resistance and thus insulin levels. It is not uncommon to find older women in their fifties and sixties with these very high levels of male hormones, so it is obvious that the menopause does not always reduce male hormone levels. This is why so many older women have a problem with facial hair and scalp hair loss.

## THYROID PROBLEMS

A deficiency of thyroid hormones can result in hair loss and dull, dry, lifeless hair. Thyroid hormone deficiency also causes the skin to become dry and more wrinkled.

| Hormone | Normal Range |
| --- | --- |
| Thyroid Stimulating Hormone | 0.2 – 4.7 mcU/ml |
| Free T4 | 4.5 – 11.2 mcg/dl |
| Free T3 | 100 – 200 ng/dl |

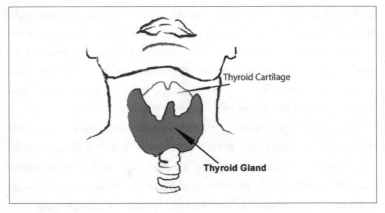

The thyroid gland often becomes underactive during the peri-menopausal years, and approximately one-third of women will develop an underactive thyroid. This may be due to shrinkage of the thyroid gland with age, or due to destruction of the thyroid gland by antibodies produced by the immune system. This is called auto-immune thyroiditis or Hashimoto's disease. The function of the thyroid gland can be tested with a simple blood test, to see if low levels of thyroid hormones are present.

The function of the thyroid gland can often be improved by taking nutritional supplements of organic selenium in a dose of 100 to 200 mcg daily. Many women will need thyroid hormone replacement therapy, which can greatly improve the hair.

Thyroid hormone replacement is available as oroxine (T4) and tertroxin (T3) tablets. Some women will need both types of thyroid hormone to restore their hair.

## GENERAL HEALTH

If you have a poor diet and unhealthy lifestyle, this will reflect in the appearance of your hair. The hair can be adversely affected by lack of sleep and stress, as these things impact upon the immune system.

Any chronic disease or auto-immune disease can adversely affect the hair, and it is well known that Lupus can be associated with hair loss. This is because the immune system produces antibodies which affect the hair follicles. Some prescription medications can cause hair loss, so check with your doctor to see if this is responsible.

### Nutritional Medicine Can Improve Your Hair

- Increase your intake of *essential fatty acids* – cold-pressed flaxseed oil, avocados, raw seeds and nuts, oily fish and cold-pressed vegetable oils and evening primrose oil.
- Take a good *multivitamin and mineral* which contains calcium, magnesium, zinc, manganese, copper, silica, selenium, B vitamins and antioxidants. Younger women or vegetarians may need a multivitamin and mineral tablet that also contains iron.
- Organic sulphur can also help the condition of the hair. Foods high in sulphur are eggs, cruciferous vegetables (cauliflower, cabbage, Brussels sprouts and broccoli) and vegetables from the onion family (onions, leeks, shallots and garlic). Some health food shops stock Vitamin C powder with organic sulphur (known as MSM), which can be mixed into fresh juices.

## JUICE RECIPE TO THICKEN YOUR HAIR

| | |
|---|---|
| 6 oz/180g | alfalfa sprouts |
| 2 | cabbage leaves or 2 Brussels sprouts |
| 6 oz/180g | broccoli florets |
| 1 | medium carrot |
| 2 | slices red onion |
| 1 | medium beet plus tops |
| 1 | clove garlic (optional) |
| 2 | slices watermelon |

Wash, trim and chop all ingredients, process through a juicer and drink immediately.

The juice improves hair because it is high in organic sulphur, phytoestrogens and the mineral silica.

According to the Women's Health Advisory Service's Trichologist and Weight Loss Consultant, Marilyn Searle, if your hair is not nourished and healthy, even the most expensive shampoos will not compensate.

## Can Oestrogen Improve My Skin?

Many women notice that their skin becomes drier and flakier after the menopause. Of course as time goes by we get more wrinkles, but this has probably got more to do with prior sun exposure, diet, hydration and smoking than it does with the menopause. However, oestrogen can definitely help to improve the texture of the skin and reduce spots. Some women tell me that their skin becomes thicker and less wrinkled after they have been on natural oestrogen and progesterone for several years. The oestrogen called oestradiol is concentrated in the deeper layers of the skin (basal epidermis). Oestrogen increases the fluid content between the skin cells and also plumps up the skin cells known as fibroblasts. Thus oestrogen therapy can improve the tone and hydration of the skin.

The amount of skin collagen declines at an average rate of 2.1

per cent per year after the menopause, irrespective of the age at which a woman goes through it. Loss of collagen in other parts of the body can result in weakened ligaments and brittle nails. Oestrogen increases collagen production in the skin and bones, which helps the skin maintain its thickness and elasticity. An adequate intake of vitamin C is very important in the maintenance of skin collagen.

### Other Techniques to Improve Your Skin

- daily use of a good cleanser and moisturizer
- a high intake of water
- regular consumption of raw vegetable and fruit juices
- supplements that contain the antioxidants selenium, zinc and vitamin E. The organic form of selenium, called selenomethionine, is best.
- supplemental flaxseed oil, which can be eaten off the spoon, added to salads or taken combined with evening primrose oil. Flaxseed oil will reduce skin dryness and improve the condition of the hair.
- avoiding excess alcohol, which can cause broken capillaries on the face
- taking special care of your liver – many skin problems such as acne rosacea, brown blemishes and inflammatory rashes and spots can be eradicated by improving liver function. The best way to support the liver is to take a good liver tonic in capsule or powder form, and to consume raw juices regularly. Organic sulphur is also beneficial for the liver, the skin and the hair. Good sources of organic sulphur are cruciferous vegetables (cabbage, broccoli, Brussels sprouts and cauliflower) and garlic, onions, shallots and leeks. You may also be able to find at a local health food shop a powder called MSM (Methyl-Sulphonyl-Methane). This powder can be taken in juices in a dose of one flat teaspoon daily.

# Chapter 11

# Special Circumstances at The Menopause

## What Can I Do after a Hysterectomy and/or Removal of My Ovaries?

The HRT requirements of a woman after a hysterectomy can vary from those of a woman who still has a uterus.

After hysterectomy the need for HRT depends upon:

- at what age the hysterectomy was done
- whether or not the ovaries were removed at the same time as the uterus – this is called an oophorectomy
- if the ovaries were not removed, whether they still working efficiently
- how severe the symptoms of hormone deficiency are
- whether the sex life been affected adversely.

If the hysterectomy was done at a relatively young age (under the age of 45), and if the ovaries are not working efficiently, then the symptoms of hormone deficiency may be quite severe. They most commonly consist of fatigue, hot flushes, disturbed sleep, dryness of the vaginal tissues, bladder problems and a large reduction in sex drive.

Initially, to relieve severe symptoms quickly an injection of oestrogen can be used. This will work within several days to relieve all these symptoms.

In the long term it is difficult to achieve stable blood levels of oestrogen with these injections, and levels tend to fluctuate from too high to too low. In such cases, implants containing natural oestrogen can be used. If depression, fatigue and sexual problems are marked, a good result can be achieved by adding an implant of testosterone along with the oestrogen implant. Generally these implants will last for 6 to 12 months, although some women tend to use up the hormones in the implant more quickly, and it can become difficult to achieve stable blood levels of hormones.

Some women who have received hormone implants require increasing doses of hormones to relieve their symptoms; it is as if their body becomes dependent upon very high blood levels of hormones. This resistance to the effect of the hormones is called *tachyphylaxis*, and can be diagnosed by finding very high levels of oestrogen and/or testosterone in blood tests, even though the patient may still be reporting symptoms of hormone deficiency. In such cases it is not safe, nor advisable, to continue using hormone implants.

For the long-term relief of symptoms after a hysterectomy and/or oophorectomy, it is safer to use hormones in the form of

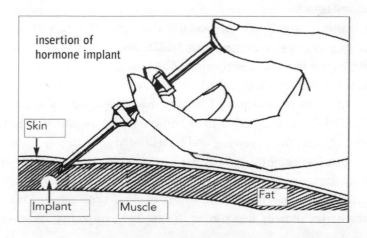

insertion of
hormone implant

Skin

Implant    Muscle

Fat

creams or lozenges. These can be tailor-made to contain any combination of natural hormones, depending upon the results of blood and/or salivary tests, and the patient's symptoms.

After a hysterectomy, many women are given only oestrogen and not any progesterone. Because natural progesterone has so many health benefits, I recommend that whenever oestrogen is prescribed, natural progesterone is always given as well. This will also avoid the hormonal imbalance of oestrogen dominance.

Some women after hysterectomy or oophorectomy complain mostly of local discomfort in the vaginal area, associated with a reduced libido and reduced ability to enjoy sexual pleasure. In these cases the use of creams containing a mixture of natural oestrogen, testosterone and progesterone can be all that is required.

DHEA can also improve the libido and increase well-being after hysterectomy. Hormonal creams are especially suitable for older women who have had a surgical menopause. These creams can be applied to the vulva and vaginal area, and generally restore sexual pleasure and function. They can be massaged into the vulva and clitoris once or twice daily.

**Case History**

Christine came to see me because she was suffering with very severe menopausal symptoms, which had started after a hysterectomy two years previously. She was now 52 years of age, and her ovaries, although still present, were no longer functional. After her hysterectomy Christine had developed a blood clot in her left leg, and had to have anti-coagulant treatment to prevent the clot from growing and travelling to her lungs.

She had recently been to her GP to ask for some hormonal help; however her GP had told her that she was unable to take any HRT because of her past history of blood clots. She had tried the herbal remedy Red Clover to ease her symptoms; however her hot flushes and vaginal dryness remained very distressing. Her blood tests revealed extremely low levels of all the sex hormones, which explained her severe symptoms.

I explained to Christine that I believed it would be safe for her to take some natural hormones in the form of a cream, which could be inserted into her vagina at night. The hormones in the creams are absorbed directly into the circulation, and do not travel to the liver until they have achieved their desired effect in the pelvic area. I did not think that Christine was at a high risk for further blood clots, as she was a fit, healthy woman and did not smoke. Christine's previous blood clot was secondary to her immobilization after surgery, and this was no longer a problem for her.

In women who form blood clots spontaneously, and for no apparent reason, we must be very careful with HRT. In these circumstances only very small amounts of transdermal hormones, using the weaker oestriol and progesterone, can be used. The same is true for women with varicose veins, when it is much safer to use transdermal creams containing only small amounts of natural hormones.

For Christine I prescribed a cream containing a mixture of oestradiol (1 mg), progesterone (20 mg) and testosterone (1 mg). I instructed her to insert half of the cream high into the vagina (with a vaginal applicator) last thing at night, and to massage the remaining half of the cream into her vulval area.

Christine was very relieved that she was able to use some form of natural HRT, as she knew that for her, the herbal treatments alone would not be adequate. So you can see that by using tailor-made natural hormone replacement therapy, we can find a programme that is suited to each woman's individual needs.

## The Menopause and Breast Cancer

All women are concerned about breast cancer and want to understand the lifestyle changes that they can make to reduce their risk. Breast cancer is the most common cancer among women, although lung cancer is the most common cause of death. Smoking cigarettes is definitely more dangerous than taking natural sex hormones; however, smoking does not receive nearly as much publicity as HRT does!

Breast cancer is rare before the age of 30, and becomes more common with age. Around two-thirds of breast cancer occurs in women aged over 50 years, and the majority occurs in women over 65. Thus women of all ages always need to examine their breasts and have regular mammograms. In the majority of older women getting breast cancer, hormonal influences are not to blame.

Several studies have shown that HRT, given for five years or more, will increase the risk of breast cancer, and many women are naturally very concerned about this. Both the WHI study and an American study reported in *The Journal of the National Cancer Institute* (vol 92, 2000, pages 328–32) show a link between oral combined HRT and breast cancer. The latter study found that there was a 10 per cent higher risk of breast cancer for every five years of HRT use. The reported ratio for breast cancer increased from 1.06 with oestrogen-only therapy to 1.24 when synthetic progestogen was added. Some researchers who are pro-HRT point out that many of these studies have design faults – they are mostly retrospective and non-randomized, and do not rule out lifestyle influences. For example, women who take HRT are generally in a higher social class, eat Western diets, drink more alcohol, have fewer children and have children at a later age. These independent risk factors for breast cancer are not generally equated for in these studies.

HRT users can take some comfort in studies such as Willis et al., published in *Cancer Causes Control* (vol 7, 1996, pages

449–57), which found that despite a slightly higher incidence of breast cancer in HRT-users, their mortality rate was 16 per cent lower. These studies have examined oral hormones (oestrogen and/or combined oestrogen and progestogen) and have not examined the effects of non-oral hormones on breast cancer risk. If oestrogen and/or synthetic progestogen increase the risk of breast cancer, then higher doses and/or more synthetic potent forms of these hormones would be expected to increase the risk the most. Conversely, small doses of natural hormones would be expected to be much safer.

If sex hormones were the major cause of breast cancer, then we could expect that EVERY woman on the planet would develop breast cancer, because all women produce sex hormones. However, breast cancer is a complex disease and many carcinogenic factors often interact to cause the cancer cells to develop. In other words, the cause of breast cancer is multi-faceted, and each contributing factor can increase the harmful effects of the others.

*Known Risk Factors for Breast Cancer*
- late menopause (after the age of 53) – produces a very slight increase.
- childbearing at a later age – women who have been pregnant at an early age create more of the weaker oestrogen, called oestriol, in their bodies. Oestriol may reduce the stimulatory effects of the more potent oestrogens (oestradiol and oestrone). This could be one of the ways that early pregnancy provides significant protection against breast cancer.
- hereditary factors – if your mother or sister had breast cancer before the menopause, you have twice the normal risk of breast cancer. The older your mother was when she got breast cancer, the lower your risk becomes. In approximately 1 in every 200 women, an inherited defective breast cancer gene is present.

- alcohol – consuming 2 drinks or more every day
- although not specifically examined, lifestyle factors that affect the immune system probably play a significant role in increasing breast cancer. The most likely ones would be a poor diet lacking in plant foods and thus phytoestrogens, deficiencies of antioxidants and selenium, smoking, and severe stress. Vegetarians have a lower risk of breast cancer, probably because they consume more phytoestrogens.

## WHAT IF YOU ARE MENOPAUSAL AND HAVE HAD BREAST CANCER?

Women who have had breast cancer, and who suffer with menopausal symptoms, need special care to:
- relieve their unpleasant symptoms of hormonal deficiency
- strengthen their immune systems to reduce the risk of the cancer recurring.

Most doctors will not feel comfortable giving prescription hormones to women with breast cancer because:
- this theoretically could increase the growth of any remaining cancer cells, especially if your cancer was positive for hormone receptors
- this could increase the likelihood of a new breast cancer occurring
- the fear of litigation, makes doctors increasingly conservative.

A significant percentage of women will suffer severe symptoms of hormone deficiency after treatment for breast cancer, especially if chemotherapy has caused a premature menopause. Probably the most common complaints are vaginal dryness and discomfort, fatigue, disturbed sleep and hot flushes.

## WHAT OPTIONS ARE AVAILABLE?

### Tamoxifen

Tamoxifen is a synthetic type of designer oestrogen, with different effects to natural oestrogen.

Tamoxifen exerts several effects:

- oestrogen-like effects upon the uterus and vagina
- anti-oestrogen-like effects upon the breast tissue.

Tamoxifen is used to treat women with breast cancer because it has been shown to reduce the recurrence rate of cancer in the opposite breast by approximately 50 per cent. Tamoxifen improves the five-year survival rate after breast cancer by approximately 25 per cent, and is generally given for up to five years after the diagnosis of breast cancer.

There is, however, a down-side to Tamoxifen:

- It increases the risk of uterine cancer (by at least 2.5 times).
- It increases the risk of blood clots (by 2 to 4 times).
- It does not relieve the symptoms of the menopause, and indeed Tamoxifen can aggravate hot flushes.

Because of the above negatives, a significant percentage of menopausal women decide not to take Tamoxifen, and prefer to rely on nutritional medicine. If Tamoxifen is producing intolerable side-effects it is probably not worth continuing with it, as it does not appear to increase survival rates with very long-term use (more than five years).

## OTHER STRATEGIES

- Vaginal gels and lubricants, which are free of hormones, can be used.
- The diet should contain an abundance of plant foods, which

contain phytoestrogens and exert an anti-cancer effect. Phytoestrogens usually reduce the symptoms of oestrogen deficiency, and improve well-being. The best foods to consume regularly are: beans of all varieties, especially soy beans and their products such as tofu and tempeh, chickpeas, lentils, alfalfa sprouts and ground flaxseeds. Other beneficial foods are vegetables, fruits, raw nuts and seeds. It is recommended that women with breast cancer obtain their phytoestrogens from their diet, and not from supplements, until more research has been done. Try to purchase organic poultry and eggs, which are free of growth-promoting hormones. Reduce your consumption of alcohol, and do not drink alcohol every day. Reduce the consumption of dairy products, as animal milks contain animal growth hormones.

- Take a good-quality antioxidant which contains organic selenium in the form of selenomethionine. The dose of organic selenium should be 100 to 200 mcg daily. Inexpensive and high-quality tablets are available that combine organic selenium with zinc and vitamins E and C.
- Drink raw juices daily – you will need to invest in a juicer. Beneficial fruits and vegetables to juice include beetroot, carrot, spinach, ginger root, dandelion leaves, red onion, cabbages of different colours, broccoli and other green leafy veg, green beans, apple, pear and pineapple. These plants contain phyto-chemicals and antioxidant nutrients, which are powerful anti-cancer agents.

## FOR WOMEN WITH BREAST CANCER WHO DECIDE TO TAKE HRT

Some women, especially young women, who have had breast cancer and suffer severely with the symptoms of a premature menopause will eventually decide to take HRT. In such young woman it can be cruel to deny any form of HRT, especially considering that the cure rate for localized breast cancer detected at an early stage is so high, so that most of these young women can expect a normal lifespan.

Some reassurance can be given to women with breast cancer who decide to take HRT from a study published in *The Journal of Clinical Oncology* in 1999. This study evaluated 319 postmenopausal women who had been free of cancer for an average of 9.5 years after treatment. In this group, 39 women decided to take oestrogen replacement, and 280 decided to avoid it. After 40 months, one woman (or 3 per cent) of the oestrogen-users developed a new breast cancer. Among the 280 women not on HRT, 14 (or 5 per cent) developed a new or recurrent cancer.

For those who are interested, Professor Cavalieri has studied the molecular origin of cancer and has found that the breakdown products of the two oestrogens oestradiol and oestrone form what are called 'oestrogen -3, 4 quinones', which can cause genetic changes that may lead to cancer, whereas oestriol does *not* form these compounds.

Conventional combined oral HRT containing oestrogen and synthetic progestogens, may increase breast cancer risk. This is why it is safer to use natural progesterone.

*Oestriol*
If a woman decides to take some form of HRT after breast cancer, theoretically it should be safer to use the weakest of all the body's oestrogens, namely oestriol. Oestriol is less likely to stimulate the breast tissues than the stronger oestradiol or oestrone. I would suggest that the use of a cream, applied to the opening of the vagina (the vulva), could be the safest option, rather than using hormone tablets. This cream could contain oestriol in a dose of 0.5 to 2 mg, combined with natural progesterone 25 to 40 mg daily. The hormones in such a cream would be taken up by the local hormone receptors in the vulva and vaginal tissues, so that less absorption into the circulation occurs.

Some experts believe that oestriol cream applied to the vulval area, is not absorbed into the bloodstream, and thus is relatively safe. This cream would relieve vaginal dryness and improve symptoms such as painful sexual intercourse and bladder problems. The small doses of hormones in such a cream would be unlikely to relieve hot flushes completely, but could certainly improve the quality of life.

Another possible alternative is to talk to your GP about the vaginal ring called ESTring, which is inserted into the vagina and is worn continuously for three months. This ring continually releases a tiny amount of oestradiol into the vagina, and can overcome vaginal dryness and discomfort. Theoretically, because the dose of oestradiol released from the ESTring is so small, it should not be absorbed into the bloodstream. Just to be sure, you can get your doctor to do a blood test for oestradiol levels after you have been using the ring or the vaginal cream for two months.

### How Can I Reduce Problems with My Bladder and Urinary System?

Urinary stress incontinence describes the lack of bladder control that some women experience when they perform actions that increase the pressure within the abdominal and pelvic cavities. This occurs when you cough, sneeze, do aerobic exercises or lift heavy objects, during which you may experience an involuntary loss of urine. Urinary Stress Incontinence (USI) is common, and affects around 25 per cent of women aged 35 and upwards; it often occurs for the first time after childbirth, or when you reach the peri-menopause. Many women are embarrassed about USI and do not seek help, preferring to live with it.

USI occurs because the muscle that closes the urethra and holds urine in the bladder (urethral sphincter), is too weak to keep the urethra closed when you do something that increases abdominal pressure. Weakness of the muscles in the bottom of the bladder, where it joins the urethra, may also contribute to

USI. If there is a prolapse – where the vaginal wall starts to descend because it has been stretched or weakened – you may also experience a lack of urinary control.

All of these problems can be made much worse by childbirth, especially if you have had a prolonged labour, or a large baby. Carrying excess weight in the abdominal area will also make the problem worse; weight loss usually results in a big improvement in USI. Heavy smoking which causes a chronic cough can also contribute to USI.

If USI comes on for the first time during the menopause, it is probably due to a deficiency of the hormone oestrogen. Lack of oestrogen causes the supporting tissues around the bladder, urethra and vagina to thin, weaken and lose their elasticity. Lack of oestrogen also increases the incidence of urinary tract infections, which will make incontinence worse.

The outer third of the urethra has oestrogen receptors, and it can become inflamed and thin without any oestrogen to keep it healthy. The best way to restore the urethra, and thus improve urinary control, is to use a small amount of an oestrogen cream every night for two weeks on the urethral area. After that time you will probably only need to apply the cream twice a week.

If you are overly sensitive to oestrogen, or want to avoid stronger oestrogens, you can ask your doctor to use the weaker oestriol in the cream, in a dose of 0.5 to 2 mg daily. Alternatively, if the oestriol cream is not strong enough, you can ask your doctor to change it to the stronger oestradiol cream.

## PELVIC FLOOR AND VAGINAL EXERCISES

These exercises can work wonders to strengthen the weakened muscles and supporting ligaments around the bladder base and urethra. These exercises are known as Kegel's exercises. Kegel's exercises have been shown to improve USI significantly in 50 to 75 per cent of cases.

### How to Do Kegel's Exercises

Contract the same muscles that you use when you voluntarily stop the flow of urine. Another way to describe Kegel's exercises is to imagine that your vagina is a lift – squeeze it in and take it up towards your navel.

To check that you are contracting the correct muscles, place two fingers in your vagina and squeeze them. Do this while keeping the abdominal muscles relaxed, and avoid pushing down. In other words, use only the vaginal muscles. Contract these muscles for 10 to 20 seconds at a time. Repeat this squeeze, 10 times, three times daily.

# Chapter 12

# How to Deal With the Side-effects of HRT

The sensitivity of individual women to possible side-effects of any hormone treatment varies greatly. This is why it is so important to tailor the correct doses and combinations of hormones for every woman.

Generally speaking, side-effects can be minimized, or overcome completely, by:

- **Using lower doses of hormones** – some women will need only very small (tiny) amounts of hormones to achieve an improvement in well-being and a resolution of unpleasant symptoms. The doses can be reduced until side-effects disappear.
- **Using different combinations of hormones** – some women will need several hormones, while others will need only one hormone, such as progesterone. If too many different types of hormones are given, some women get too much interaction between the hormones, or the action of one hormone becomes too predominant. Thus in women who get heavy bleeding, natural progesterone only would be prescribed, and oestrogen avoided. Women who find that their HRT is not helping their sex life may need higher doses of natural testosterone. If HRT

causes acne, then testosterone would be stopped, and only DHEA and natural oestrogen and progesterone would be used.

- **Using natural hormones** – structurally identical to the body's naturally produced hormones; these are called 'bio-identical hormones'. These natural hormones do not block the body's hormone receptors from the action of other hormones. The synthetic hormones are more likely to cause side-effects because they are more difficult for the liver to break down.
- **Using hormones that do not get absorbed from the gut.** This is because oral hormones, after absorption from the gut, pass straight to the liver. The liver is designed to break down these hormones so that smaller amounts than were ingested actually get into the circulation. Thus, higher doses of hormones are needed to compensate for this liver breakdown. The oral hormones also have a much greater chance of causing metabolic changes in the liver, such as an increased production of clotting factors. Oral hormones, especially in high doses, increase the workload of the detoxification pathways in the liver.

## Solutions to side-effects from HRT

| HORMONE SIDE-EFFECT | SUGGESTED SOLUTION |
| --- | --- |
| Acne, pimples, facial hair and greasy skin. Hair loss from the scalp | Avoid masculine progestogens such as norethindrone, and use cyproterone acetate, or natural progesterone instead. Reduce the dose of testosterone and DHEA, or stop using these hormones. Increase the dose of oestrogen. |
| Weight gain | Avoid oral forms of HRT. Avoid synthetic progesterones. Reduce doses of all hormones, especially testosterone. |

| HORMONE SIDE-EFFECT | SUGGESTED SOLUTION |
|---|---|
| Breast swelling and tenderness | Reduce the dose of oestrogen, or change to a weaker oestrogen such as oestriol. Include natural progesterone. |
| Heavy menstrual bleeding, period cramps, increased size of fibroids, aggravation of endometriosis | Stop or reduce the dose of oestrogen or change to a weaker oestrogen such as oestriol. Increase the dose of natural progesterone. |
| Increase in blood pressure, aching legs, fluid retention, leg cramps | Stop or reduce the dose of oestrogen or change to a weaker oestrogen such as oestriol. Use oestrogen creams or patches and not troches or tablets. Avoid synthetic progesterones. |
| High cholesterol | Avoid synthetic progesterones and change to natural progesterone. Avoid testosterone. |
| Migraine headaches, nausea and vomiting | Reduce the dose of oestrogen and avoid oral oestrogens. Use oestrogen creams or patches in small doses only. Avoid synthetic progestogens. |
| Blood clots | Avoid oral oestrogen and use only very small doses of the weaker oestrogens such as oestriol. Use only transdermal oestrogens, such as creams or patches. Avoid synthetic progestogens, and only use natural progesterone creams. |
| Aggravation of gall stones | Avoid oral oestrogens and use small doses of oestrogen in creams and patches containing the weaker oestrogen called oestriol. |
| Spotting and breakthrough bleeding | Stop the HRT until bleeding ceases completely, and then recommence the HRT using half the prescribed dose. If bleeding recurs, reduce the dose of oestrogen. Change to oestrogen creams or patches. You may need to increase the dose of progesterone. See your gynaecologist if irregular and/or heavy bleeding persists, as it may be due to a growth in the uterus. |

## Bleeding and HRT

If you are taking HRT and you still have a uterus, you need to decide if you want to avoid menstrual bleeding or if you want to have a regular monthly bleed. It is the progesterone component of the HRT that causes the bleed, as it causes the uterine lining that has been built up by the oestrogen to shed itself. If you do not want to experience any bleeding, this can usually be achieved by taking progesterone every day along with the oestrogen. If you take progesterone every day, then generally a smaller dose of progesterone can be used. For 8 out of 10 women who use progesterone continuously, periods will stop. You may have some light spotting or a minor period during the first three months of taking both hormones continuously, then the bleeding usually gradually ceases completely.

For women who want to have a monthly bleed, the progesterone is given cyclically, so that it is taken for 10 to 14 days of every calendar month. Sometimes women who take progesterone cyclically along with their oestrogen will not have any bleeding at all. This is nothing to worry about. It just means that you are not taking enough oestrogen to cause the uterine lining to build up, so there is no lining to shed.

All women with a uterus who are taking oestrogen must take progesterone to prevent over-stimulation of the uterine lining. Generally speaking, your bleeding will be lighter while on HRT, compared to the amount of menstrual bleeding you had before the menopause. Some women stop HRT because they cannot put up with the annoyance of bleeding, however by lowering the dose of oestrogen, or increasing the amount of progesterone, we can often avoid any bleeding.

While on cyclical HRT your bleeding pattern should become regular, and bleeding will generally commence within two to three days after stopping the progesterone. This regular bleeding pattern should reproduce itself every month, provided you have not missed taking your hormones regularly. If your bleeding becomes irregular, prolonged or heavy while you are taking HRT, you must tell your doctor. This is because the bleeding could be due to physical problems such as polyps in the uterus or cervix, fibroids, hyperplasia of the uterine lining, or even the early stages of cancer. Usually the bleeding is nothing serious; however do not delay in seeing your gynaecologist. The gynaecologist will do a thorough pelvic examination and an ultrasound scan of the pelvis to check for any physical problems. The ultrasound scan will display the thickness of the uterine lining (endometrium); if it is less than 6 mm thick, it is not hyperplasia. Your gynaecologist may also want to do an endometrial biopsy to check the cells lining the uterus.

If you experience irregular or heavy bleeding stop the HRT until the bleeding ceases completely. If you have to wait a few weeks before you can see the gynaecologist and your symptoms return, you can recommence the HRT using half the previous dose.

Hopefully your gynaecologist will not find any physical reason for the bleeding, in which case the bleeding is occurring because the balance of your HRT is wrong for you. Talk to your doctor about readjusting your dose of hormones to regulate your bleeding or to avoid breakthrough bleeding altogether.

Some women continue to get a light period, or some breakthrough bleeding, for several years after commencing HRT. Generally speaking, as you get older the bleeding will get lighter and lighter, and eventually disappear completely. Some women worry when their periods disappear, but this is nothing to be concerned about. It just means that the amount of oestrogen that you are taking is not enough to produce a significant lining inside the uterus. So if there is no lining, there is nothing to shed, and thus no periods will occur.

### Case History
Catherine had been using a prescription hormonal cream for six months to help her with menopausal symptoms. Her cream

contained a daily dose of Triest (see page 74) 2 mg, progesterone 50 mg and testosterone 3 mg. She was very pleased with the effect of this cream, because it had relieved her hot flushes and increased her energy levels. It had also helped her libido and had made her feel desirable and attractive.

However, she had gained 4 kg (10 pounds) and had experienced some spots on her face since she had been on this cream, and came to see me as she was not happy about the weight gain.

I did a blood test to check her hormone levels, and found that her Free Androgen Index (FAI) was elevated above normal levels. This was due to the relatively high amount of testosterone in her cream, so I changed her prescription so that she was receiving only 0.5 mg of testosterone daily in her cream. Over the next three months, Catherine found that her spots cleared up and her weight returned to normal.

This case history illustrates how excessive amounts of testosterone can lead to weight gain and spots. Many women find that once the natural HRT has corrected their symptoms, they can have their prescription changed to provide a lower daily dose of hormones. By adjusting the doses as needed to correct the symptoms, we are able to use the lowest necessary dose of hormones, and are able to avoid side-effects.

**Case History**

Juliane was 55 years of age and had been taking a combined tablet containing the hormones oestradiol and norethisterone for three years to relieve her menopausal symptoms.

She had found this helped to clear up her hot flushes and fatigue, but felt it was not quite correct for her. She had noticed some hair loss from the top and sides of her scalp, increasing facial hair, weight gain and spots on her chin. Juliane weighed 72 kg (11 stone 3) and was carrying most of the excess weight in her abdomen.

I explained to Juliane that the synthetic progestogen in her HRT tablet had a slightly androgenic effect, and acted like a weak male hormone as well as a progestogen.

Juliane's blood tests did not reveal any gross abnormalities, and her FAI was normal, because the oral hormones had increased her levels of Sex Hormone Binding Globulin (SHBG). However, the norethisterone in her HRT tablet was too masculine for her body; this was why she was getting the male hormone-like side-effects.

After some discussion I changed her prescription to oestradiol tablets and cyproterone tablets. The cyproterone would act as an anti-androgen and make her hormonal profile more feminine. This worked as expected and, 12 months later, Juliane had lost the excess weight and her skin and hair were back to normal. She had been following the Syndrome X eating plan (see pages 115–22) and was eating more protein and salads to correct her metabolism. Now that she was getting older, she wanted to change to a lower dose of HRT, so we changed her prescription to a cream containing natural Triest 2 mg and natural progesterone 50 mg daily. She did not need any testosterone, as this would cause her hair loss to recur.

You can see that the prescription of hormones for the menopause needs to be regularly reviewed, as it may need changing over the passage of time. Generally speaking, in older women the aim is to use the lowest dose of natural hormones that works well to relieve the symptoms and maintain a physiological balance of hormones.

# Chapter 13

# How Can I Reduce the Risk of Osteoporosis?

Osteoporosis means loss of bone mass, and results in bone fragility. Osteoporosis is very common, affecting 50 per cent women over 60. Statistics show that for women entering the menopause, the lifelong risk of hip fracture is around 15 per cent, which is equal to the combined risk of breast, ovarian and uterine cancer.

Osteoporosis of the spine

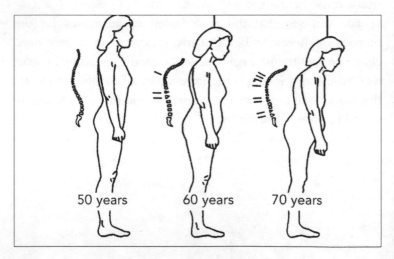

50 years     60 years     70 years

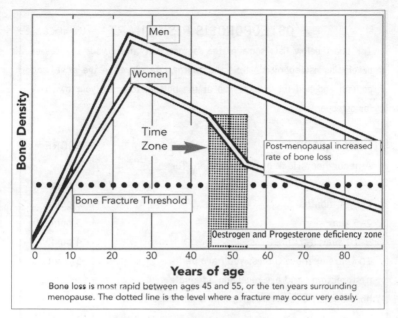

Bone loss is most rapid between ages 45 and 55, or the ten years surrounding menopause. The dotted line is the level where a fracture may occur very easily.

The increasing risk of bone fracture with the menopause

You can see that the time zone around the menopause, represented by the shaded column in the graph above, is a crucial time-corridor where the loss of bone mass can be greatly accelerated. Indeed, because of the loss of oestrogen during this time, a rapid bone-loser can lose a large amount of her total bone mass. More than 50 per cent of the total amount of bone that is lost in the postmenopausal years is usually lost in the first seven to ten years after the menopause.

# OSTEOPOROSIS RISK CHART

The chart below lists some of the factors that affect your chances of developing osteoporosis. Circle the appropriate scores in the right-hand column and add the numbers up at the bottom to score your own risk for osteoporosis.

| RISK FACTOR | SCORE |
|---|---|
| Amenorrhoea (lack of menstruation) for: | |
| 6–12 months | 1 point |
| 12–24 months | 2 points |
| 2–5 years | 3 points |
| 5–10 years | 4 points |
| 10 years or more (unless you have had a hysterectomy and are receiving adequate hormone replacement therapy, in which case score 0) | 5 points |
| | |
| First menstrual period after the age of 17 (late puberty) | 1 point |
| Long term use of cortisone | 5 points |
| Family history of osteoporosis | 3 points |
| Small, fine-boned frame | 2 points |
| Calcium deficiency during adolescence and/or while nursing a child | 2 points |
| Tobacco use | 1 point |
| Lack of weight-bearing exercise | 2 points |
| Excessive exercise, especially if it leads to amenorrhoea | 2 points |
| Caucasian or Asian racial background | 1 point |
| Excessive consumption of salt, alcohol, caffeine, soft drinks | 1 point |
| Overactive thyroid (excess thyroxine) | 1 point |
| TOTAL SCORE | |

If your total score is under 5 on this scale, you have a low risk of developing osteoporosis.

If your total score is 5 to 8 points, you have a moderate risk of developing osteoporosis.

If your total score is 9 or more points, you have a high risk of developing osteoporosis.

The most accurate test for measuring the bone mineral density, and thus the strength of your bones, is called the DEXA scan. DEXA stands for Dual Energy X-ray Absorptiometry, and this test accurately measures bone mineral density in the hip, spine or wrist. A DEXA test is easy and quick to perform, and exposes you to only a tiny amount of radiation. Standard X-rays are not a very sensitive indicator of bone loss, and may not reveal osteo-porosis until you have lost 20 to 30 per cent of your bone mass, which is way too late to discover you are losing bone. In contrast, the very sensitive DEXA test can detect very small and early amounts of bone loss of around only 1 to 2 per cent. The lower the bone mineral density, the higher the risk of bone fractures.

Now that combined oral HRT is no longer to be prescribed routinely on a long-term basis for the prevention of osteoporo-sis, women need to be informed about other ways of building and maintaining their bone density.

**The best way to maintain a good bone density is to exercise reg-ularly. This has been proven to slow bone loss.**
A good exercise routine would consist of exercising for 40 to 60 minutes daily, with a combination of:
- walking
- lifting light weights, which can be done while walking or doing aqua-aerobics
- golf, tennis, netball or aqua aerobics
- dancing – you can even do this at home to some nice boppy

music and use a pair of hand weights while you dance
- joining a local gym and learning a graduated set of exercises
- getting a personal trainer if you lack motivation
- yoga and/or tai chi

**Exercises to improve balance** are very important because most fractures occur during a fall, and women are far more likely to fall if they have poor balance and poor co-ordination. The best exercises to improve balance and co-ordination are yoga and tai chi. Regular exercise builds muscle strength, which is just as important as bone strength, because if you fall the muscles will contract to prevent excessive flexion of the joints and bones. Many women fracture bones not because of poor bone density, but because they have poor muscle strength and poor balance, which makes them susceptible to frequent falls. Regular muscle-building exercises and tai chi or yoga can make you as sure-footed as a mountain goat! If there were no falls, there would be no hip or forearm fractures.

## Mineral Supplements

These should be started at least 10 years before the menopause, because the loss of bone during the 10 years before the menopause is often quite marked. It is important to take minerals every day to ensure that your bones are receiving adequate amounts; most women are mineral deficient and, let's be honest – do you have a perfect diet? Very few people have, and even if your diet is good you probably have had a mineral-deficient diet at some stage of your life. Processed foods are very low in minerals, and the soil foods are grown in have become increasingly deficient in the trace and macro-minerals needed for strong bones.

The latest information shows that most women (and men) do not get enough calcium in the diet. Adequate calcium and mineral intake can greatly slow down the rate of post-menopausal bone loss, and will reduce fracture rates.

A good mineral supplement to reduce osteoporosis should contain:

- calcium citrate and calcium hydroxyapatite – these types of calcium are well absorbed and utilized
- zinc, manganese, copper, silica and magnesium – essential minerals that help calcium to strengthen the bones, cartilage and connective tissues.

## VITAMIN D

Vitamin D deficiency is common in women who do not spend much time outdoors, women who have a low-fat diet, women with digestive problems and women who smoke and/or eat poorly. It is easy to check the levels of vitamin D (serum 25-hydroxyvitamin D3) with a simple blood test. In women with low bone density, or multiple risk factors for osteoporosis, I always check the blood levels of vitamin D. If they are found to be low, it is essential to supplement with vitamin D, as this vitamin is required for efficient absorption and utilization of calcium.

## DRUGS USED TO BUILD AND MAINTAIN BONE DENSITY

These may be prescribed by a doctor, and consist of:
*Calcitriol*
This is a synthetic form of vitamin D which increases calcium absorption from the gut and reduces calcium excretion, resulting in a positive calcium balance in the body. Calcitriol is a more active form of vitamin D, compared to the regular vitamin D found in supplements or the diet.

The dose of Calcitriol is 0.25 mcg twice daily in capsule form. Calcitriol has been proven to maintain and even increase bone formation, and can reduce fractures. Calcitriol is a treatment for post-menopausal women who have diagnosed osteoporosis. Calcitriol is generally very well tolerated, and has very few, and only infrequent, side-effects. The most common side-effect is raised blood calcium, which can result in nausea, headaches or weakness. These side-effects can be quickly overcome after reducing calcium intake and stopping the medication, after which smaller doses may be required.

Calcium and vitamin D supplements should not be taken while you are on Calcitriol.

*Bisphosphonates*

Like HRT, bisphosphonates prevent bone loss. Bisphosphonates have been proven to reduce bone loss and increase bone building. The best known examples are Etidronate (Didronel) and Alendronate (Fosamax). Fosamax is very effective and has been shown to reduce hip fractures by 56 per cent and spinal fractures by 49 per cent in women who have osteoporosis. The bisphosphonate drugs can have unpleasant side-effects upon the digestive tract, and may cause severe indigestion and heartburn. To avoid these problems, they should be taken with 250 ml of water on an empty stomach, first thing in the morning. You must then remain upright for 30 minutes, with no drink or food. The effectiveness of Fosamax is increased by taking it with either raloxifene (see below) or HRT, although HRT is not recommended for long-term use (over five years).

*SERMs*

Raloxifene is an example of a SERM (Selective Oestrogen Receptor Modulator). SERMs are a new generation of synthetic oestrogens (designer oestrogens) which can be used in post-menopausal women who have low bone density. Raloxifene is able to reduce osteoporosis, but does not increase bone mass as much as real oestrogen or Fosamax.

Although raloxifene is a new drug, it does not appear to increase the risk of breast or uterine cancer at this stage of our knowledge. Unlike natural or equine oestrogens, raloxifene does not stimulate oestrogen receptors in the breast or uterus. Because it is a selective oestrogen, it is often prescribed for women with osteoporosis who are also at risk for breast cancer. Raloxifene is prescribed in a dose of one tablet daily. It does not relieve other menopausal symptoms such as hot flushes or vaginal dryness.

The SERM drugs are known to increase the risk of blood clots occurring in the deep veins, and should be avoided in women with varicose veins or a past history of blood clots. These drugs cannot be prescribed in women with liver disease, as they must be broken down by the liver. Side-effects of raloxifene include hot flushes, vaginal dryness, headaches, weight gain and leg cramps.

### Osteoporosis and Tooth loss

Tooth loss for no apparent reason, which may be associated with periodontal disease, can be a sign of underlying osteoporosis. Studies have shown that women with osteoporosis who still have their natural teeth at age 50, will have a greater chance (44 per cent) of needing full dentures by age 60, whereas only 15 per cent of women who do not have osteoporosis will require dentures by this age. This loss of teeth is due to loss of bone in the jaw, which allows the gums to become diseased and loose; this bone loss can be detected by X-ray of the jaws. If you have loss of bone in the jaws, you are probably losing bone in other parts of the skeleton. The use of regular mineral supplements can reduce this bone loss in the jaw, and thus prevent tooth loss. Vitamin C, citrus fruits and apples are good for the gums and connective tissues, which hold the teeth in place.

Many different foods contain calcium, but some contain more than others. The Table below will give you an idea of which foods are the best sources of calcium. Use it to see whether your normal diet is providing you with the recommended 1,000 mg of calcium per day. If not, you should either include more calcium-rich foods in your diet or take supplemental calcium to make sure you get enough of this vital mineral.

| FOOD | SERVING SIZE | CALCIUM (mg) |
|------|--------------|--------------|
| **DAIRY PRODUCTS** | | |
| Buttermilk | 240ml / 8fl oz | 285 |
| Cheese | | |
|     Camembert | 30g / 1 oz | 110 |
|     Cheddar | 30g / 1 oz | 204 |
|     cottage | 115g / 4 oz | 135 |
|     cream | 30g / 1 oz | 23 |
|     feta | 30g / 1 oz | 140 |
|     mozzarella, part-skim | 30g / 1 oz | 207 |
|     Muenster | 30g / 1 oz | 203 |
|     Parmesan, grated | 1 tablespoon | 69 |
|     ricotta, part skim | 60g / 2 oz | 335 |
|     Jarlsberg | 30g / 1 oz | 219 |
| Cow's Milk | | |
|     low-fat (2 per cent) | 240ml / 8 fl oz | 297 |
|     skim | 240ml / 8 floz | 302 |
|     skim, powdered | 1 tablespoon | 130 |
|     whole | 240ml / 8 fl oz | 291 |
| Egg | 1 large | 25 |
| Goat's milk | 240ml / 8 fl oz | 350 |
| Sour cream | 1 tablespoon | 16 |
| Yoghurt, plain | | |
|     whole-milk | 240ml / 8 fl oz | 275 |
|     nonfat-milk | 240ml / 8 fl oz | 452 |
| **FISH** | | |
| Clams, tinned | 90g / 3 oz | 78 |
| Crabmeat, tinned | 90g / 3 oz | 38 |

| FOOD | SERVING SIZE | CALCIUM (mg) |
|---|---|---|
| Flounder or sole, baked | 90g / 3 oz | 16 |
| Haddock, grilled | 90g / 3 oz | 51 |
| Oysters | 115g / 4 oz | 111 |
| Salmon. pink, tinned | 90g / 3 oz | 181 |
| Sardines, tinned, drained | 90g / 3 oz | 325 |
| Prawns or scallops, cooked | 90g / 3 oz | 39 |
| Tuna, light, tinned | 90g / 3 oz | 10 |
| **NUTS AND SEEDS** | | |
| Almonds, unsalted | 30g / 1 oz | 70 |
| Brazil nuts, unsalted | 30g / 1 oz | 55 |
| Pistachio nuts, unsalted | 30g / 1 oz | 40 |
| Sesame seeds, ground | 30g / 1 oz | 290 |
| Sunflower seeds | 30g / 1 oz | 30 |
| Walnuts, unsalted | 30g / 1 oz | 30 |
| Tahini | 1 tablespoon | 85 |
| **LEGUMES AND SOY PRODUCTS** | | |
| Baked beans | 115g / 4 oz | 60 |
| Chickpeas | 115g / 4 oz | 75 |
| Hummus | 1 tablespoon | 15 |
| Kidney beans | 90g / 3 oz | 60 |
| Lima Beans | 90g / 3 oz | 40 |
| Miso | 115g / 4 oz | 92 |
| Peanuts, roasted | 90g / 3 oz | 54 |
| Peanut butter | 1 tablespoon | 6 |
| Refried beans, tinned | 90g / 3 oz | 59 |
| Soy milk | 240ml / 8 fl oz | 10 |
| Soy milk, calcium enriched | 240ml / 8 fl oz | 300 |

| FOOD | SERVING SIZE | CALCIUM (mg) |
|---|---|---|
| Soybeans, cooked | 115g / 4 oz | 90 |
| Tofu | 145g / 5 oz | 130 |
| | | |
| **FRUITS** | 1 medium | 10 |
| Apple | 200g / 7 oz | 100 |
| Apricots, dried, uncooked | 1 medium | 26 |
| Avocado | 1 medium | 7 |
| Banana | 140g / 5 oz | 46 |
| Blackberries, raw | 140g / 5 oz | 9 |
| Blueberries, fresh, raw | ½ medium | 29 |
| Cantaloupe | 10 medium | 27 |
| Dates, whole, pitted | 10 medium | 269 |
| Figs, dried | ½ medium | 14 |
| Grapefruit | 10 medium | 5 |
| Grapes, seedless | 1 medium | 20 |
| Kiwi fruit | 1 medium | 21 |
| Mango | 1 medium | 30 |
| Orange | 1 medium | 72 |
| Papaya | 1 medium | 4 |
| Peach | 1 medium | 20 |
| Pear | 200g / 7 oz | 11 |
| Pineapple, fresh, cubed | 10 medium | 43 |
| Prunes, uncooked | 115g / 4 oz | 27 |
| Raspberries | 75g / 2½ oz | 170 |
| Rhubarb, cooked | 140g / 5 oz | 27 |
| Strawberries | 10-cm wedge | 30 |
| Watermelon | | |
| | | |
| **VEGETABLES** | | |
| Asparagus, fresh, cooked | 90g / 3 oz | 22 |

| FOOD | SERVING SIZE | CALCIUM (mg) |
|---|---|---|
| Beets | 90g / 3 oz | 15 |
| Broccoli, fresh, cooked | 1 medium spear | 83 |
| Brussels sprouts, fresh, cooked | 60g / 2 oz | 28 |
| Bok choy, fresh, raw | 30g / 1 oz | 37 |
| Cabbage, raw | 60g / 2 oz | 32 |
| Cabbage, cooked, drained | 90g / 3 oz | 50 |
| Carrots, fresh, raw | 1 medium | 19 |
| Carrots, fresh, cooked | 75g / 2½ oz | 24 |
| Cauliflower, fresh, cooked | 75g / 2½ oz | 17 |
| Celery, fresh, raw | 1 medium stalk | 16 |
| Collard greens, cooked | 30g / 1 oz | 27 |
| Green beans, fresh, cooked | 60g / 2 oz | 29 |
| Kale, fresh, cooked | 30g / 1 oz | 47 |
| Mustard greens, cooked | 30g / 1 oz | 76 |
| Onions | | |
|    raw | 1 medium | 30 |
|    cooked | 90g / 3 oz | 23 |
| Peas, green, cooked | 90g / 3 oz | 19 |
| Potato,baked, with skin | 1 medium | 20 |
| Pumpkin, canned | 115g / 4 oz | 64 |
| Sauerkraut | 115g / 4 oz | 36 |
| Spinach | | |
|    raw, fresh | 30g / 1 oz | 27 |
|    cooked, drained | 115g / 4 oz | 130 |
| Squash, acorn or butternut, mashed | 115g / 4 oz | 52 |
| Sweet potato, cooked | 1 medium | 32 |
| Tomato | 1 medium | 6 |
| Zucchini, cooked | 75g / 2½ oz | 12 |

| FOOD | SERVING SIZE | CALCIUM (mg) |
| --- | --- | --- |
| **GRAINS AND GRAIN PRODUCTS** | | |
| Barley, cooked | 170g / 6 oz | 17 |
| Bulgur, cooked | 170g / 6 oz | 18 |
| Bread, most types | 1 slice | 0 |
| Breakfast cereal, most types | 90g / 3 oz | 5–30 |
| Muesli, homemade | 115g / 4 oz | 76 |
| Oatmeal, cooked | 90g / 3 oz | 19 |
| Pasta, enriched, cooked | 140g / 5 oz | 10 |
| Rice, brown, cooked | 170g / 6 oz | 20 |
| Rice, white enriched, cooked | 170g / 6 oz | 23 |
| **MISCELLANEOUS** | 1 teaspoon | 32 |
| Basil, ground | 1 teaspoon | 38 |
| Celery seed | 30g / 1 oz | 50 |
| Chocolate, milk, plain | 1 teaspoon | 28 |
| Cinnamon | | |
| Molasses | 1 tablespoon | 137 |
| blackstrap | 1 tablespoon | 12 |
| Sugar, brown | | |

# Chapter 14

# Depression and Anxiety During the Menopause

It is well known that mood disorders are more common during the peri-menopausal years, and I personally see a lot of depressed and/or anxious menopausal women.

## What Are Some of the Causes of Depression in These Women?

- The loss of sex hormones can affect the level of the brain chemicals known as neuro-transmitters. The loss of the steroid sex hormones may cause a reduction of the brain chemicals called serotonin and of the biogenic amines, which influence mood, appetite, sleep and sex drive. There are receptors in the brain for oestrogen, progesterone and testosterone.
- There may be a sense of loss associated with ageing and the end of fertility – this could relate to children leaving home, a loss of sexuality, a loss of youth, or a change in career. It is not uncommon for marriages and relationships to falter or change during the peri-menopausal years.
- There may be increased stress levels, which commonly result from dealing with problematic teenagers or ailing ageing

parents. This can increase responsibilities and workload to unacceptably high levels. The straw that breaks the camel's back may lead to a stress breakdown, which then results in a depressive illness or panic attacks.

- Genetic factors are always significant, and there may be a family history of depressive illness.

The use of natural HRT can achieve an improvement in moods and make you feel more energetic, feminine and desirable.

Testosterone increases energy and mental drive, and can make you feel more confident.

Oestrogen often improves the quality of sleep, and this can reduce depression and anxiety. Oestrogen can also tone down aggression and make you feel more cheery. Too much oestrogen, however, can make you feel too passive and yielding.

Natural progesterone can make you feel more relaxed and easy going; some people have referred to progesterone as 'the happy hormone'.

Some women get a complete relief of mood disorders from HRT, and are not willing to give it up for these reasons.

If your depression is due to sexual problems and/or poor communication with your partner, then HRT can be very helpful in overcoming these problems. Don't forget to have the hormone levels of your partner checked as well, if there are problems with poor libido and lack of interest.

## NATURAL SUBSTANCES THAT CAN HELP

- St John's Wort
- magnesium – I call magnesium 'the great relaxer'
- vitamin B complex
- essential fatty acids from cold-pressed-flaxseed oil and oily fish, raw nuts and seeds

These supplements can make a big difference, not only to your moods but also to your memory and mental ability. You need to be regular in taking them, and they may take four to six weeks to make a big difference, so patience is needed.

- Exercise and increasing your fitness level will also reduce depression and anxiety, as well as improve sleep. This is because the levels of the brain's natural happy chemicals (endorphins), as well as Growth Hormone levels, are increased by regular exercise.

## IF THE ANXIETY IS SEVERE

If anxiety is severe and is associated with insomnia and/or panic attacks, a tricyclic anti-depressant drug may work wonders. The tricyclic drugs are very effective, and in small doses are usually free of significant side-effects. They are not habit forming, which is nice to know, and is in contrast with the sedative drugs such as Valium, Xanax, etc., which are often very difficult to stop taking. Side-effects of the tricyclic drugs may include a dry mouth, blurred vision and morning drowsiness; however these side-effects usually disappear after the first two weeks of use.

## IF THERE IS DEPRESSION AS WELL AS ANXIETY

If depression and anxiety are present, the modern-day class of anti-depressants known as the Selective Serotonin Re-uptake Inhibitors (SSRIs) can be extremely effective. These drugs increase the amount of serotonin in the brain, and are powerful anti-depressants. The SSRIs can also reduce anxiety and promote a deep restful sleep. Possible side-effects of the SSRIs are a reduction in sex drive, inability to have orgasms and slight drowsiness, although the latter side-effect is uncommon. Although the SSRIs are not addictive, it can take time to come off them, and a gradual reduction in dosage over several months is recommended, to avoid a recurrence of depressive symptoms. In those with a severe depressive illness, or a very stressful ongoing life situation, it is usually best to continue the SSRIs for several years or even longer, to be able to achieve a good quality of life.

## How Do I Know If I Need an Anti-depressant?

This is a difficult question, and is ideally worked out after you have had some time with a professional counsellor or a doctor who is interested in counselling.

At the Women's Health Advisory Service in Sydney we get hundreds of phone calls from women who are having emotional difficulties and trouble coping with life changes during the menopause. We also receive quite a few calls from caring husbands and partners who are at a loss in how to help the woman in their life. Yes, it is important to have someone to call and chat with, however it takes time, objectivity and skill to work out the deepest feelings and the psycho-dynamics of your subconscious mind. This is where a professional counsellor, psychologist or therapist is able to help you enormously.

For example, if you feel depressed and unhappy, it could be due to:

- an unhappy marriage or relationship that is emotionally toxic for you
- a deep insecurity that prevents you from leaving an unhappy relationship
- poor self-esteem that prevents you from growing in yourself
- inability to let go of past or present negative experiences
- trying to change your partner or a family member when this is impossible; far better to devote your time and energies to yourself
- unrealistic expectations of life
- coping with ageing and sick parents

- inability to find fulfilment after the children leave home
- a feeling of losing your identity
- poor health and fatigue due to hidden illness
- a chemical imbalance in your brain.

When you are unhappy within yourself then nothing seems right around you, and your sense of judgement becomes clouded; in other words, you cannot be objective about yourself. When depression is effectively treated, people find that they can then see things more clearly and make the right decisions. While you are depressed, or besieged with other negative emotions, you may make decisions that you regret later. For example, sometimes women will tell us that, in hindsight, they regret leaving their marriage or relationship. Conversely, other women will benefit from leaving a relationship and just concentrating on improving themselves mentally and physically. Some women may make bad business decisions and give up years of hard work, just because they are depressed. It is not wise to make major decisions while you are still depressed; get effective treatment of your depression first, before making these big decisions.

The good news is that with modern-day anti-depressant drugs, a depressive illness is usually alleviated within four to six weeks of beginning the medication.

A good counsellor will explore all these issues with you, and this may be all that you need to lift yourself out of the clouds of depression and confusion. If counselling and support do not help you, then you are far more likely to need an anti-depressant medication.

### Will the Menopause Affect My Memory?

Our memory can be affected by many things, including:

- depression and anxiety
- poor concentration and inability to stop our thoughts from distracting us

- lack of sleep and fatigue
- poor diet
- drug misuse, such as excessive smoking and excess alcohol
- an excess intake of some medications, such as sleeping tablets, pain killers and some anti-inflammatory drugs
- hormonal imbalances during the menopause
- degenerative diseases of the brain.

The memory can almost always be restored by correcting the above causes, but of course the third time you put the keys in the fridge and can't recall a word, you secretly worry that you may be in the early stages of Alzheimer's disease. Dementia increases with ageing, so one would think that if hormone therapy is responsible for an increased lifespan, there would be a higher incidence of dementia in women taking long-term oestrogen. However, this has not been found to be the case. In a study sample of New Yorkers where Alzheimer's dementia was present in around 16 per cent of elderly women, the incidence of Alzheimer's disease was decreased to 5.8 per cent among the women on HRT.

I have noticed that women who start on natural progesterone often tell me that their memory has improved. The natural hormone called pregnenolone can also improve memory and moods.

## NUTRITIONAL THERAPIES TO IMPROVE MEMORY

- Ensure adequate hydration with pure water and raw juices, to provide plentiful anti-oxidants to prevent free radicals from damaging your brain cells. Elevated homocysteine levels in the brain have been associated with Alzheimer's disease. Homocysteine is a protein, present in the blood, which is toxic in high amounts; the best way to reduce the toxic homocysteine is to increase folic acid intake. Raw vegetables are the best source of folic acid, so as far as your brain is concerned, it pays to juice!

- Increase your intake of essential omega-3 fatty acids in the diet, found in cold-pressed flaxseed oil, oily fish, organic eggs, raw nuts and seeds.
- Take an anti-oxidant containing organic selenium (selenomethionine), vitamin E and vitamin C to protect your brain against free radicals.
- Keep your liver healthy, as it is the filter and cleanser of the bloodstream, and removes the dangerous fat-soluble toxins that can accumulate in your brain. The brain is largely composed of fat, and thus is a repository for fat-soluble toxins which only the liver can break down and eliminate.
- Avoid exposure to petrochemicals (see page 51) as these are fat-soluble toxins, which accumulate in the brain.
- Take regular exercise to improve the circulation of blood to the brain cells.
- Eat first-class protein three times daily, as the brain's neurotransmitters are made from amino acids. Many women do not eat enough regular protein, and thus lack the essential amino acids.
- Take a supplement of magnesium, which is required for over 300 enzyme systems in the body, including many in the brain.
- You may find that herbs such as gingko biloba, bilberry and garlic improve the peripheral and cerebral circulation.
- Perform regular mental exercises, such as activities which require planning and logic, crosswords, reading or intellectual games. The brain is like a muscle – if you do not use the neural pathways regularly, they will become sluggish and lazy.

## How Can I Improve My Sleep?

Menopausal women troubled by nocturnal hot flushes and sweating will benefit from the use of natural oestrogen. This can be given as a patch or cream, or indeed in any way that your doctor and you decide is best. The cream can be rubbed into the skin or the vulva on retiring.

For those wanting to avoid all forms of HRT, the herbs sage and hops can help, and can be drunk as herbal teas or taken in tincture form.

## OTHER TIPS FOR IMPROVING SLEEP

- Go to bed when you become tired – and do *not* watch TV in bed.
- Avoid eating sugar or refined carbohydrates during the two hours before retiring, as these may destabilize blood sugar levels. If you are hungry, have a protein snack such as some tinned fish or cottage cheese and fruit, before retiring.
- Do not drink large amounts of fluids in the evening, to prevent frequent visits to the bathroom, and avoid caffeine after lunchtime.
- Avoid alcohol, because it is known to reduce the secretion of melatonin. Alcohol also interferes with the REM sleep, which is required for dreaming, and inhibits the deepest phase of sleep called the delta phase.
- Do not watch the clock!
- Take walks in the sunlight – exposure to bright sunlight in the morning will influence the pineal gland to secrete melatonin earlier in the evening.
- Half an hour before sleep, get yourself into a relaxed mode – have a hot bath and listen to relaxing music. Meditation techniques can help to put your brainwave patterns into a mode that is conducive to sleep. Listening to your breath as it is going in and out, while rejecting vexatious thoughts, can be a powerful relaxant upon the mind.
- If you live in a noisy area, you can soundproof your room with dark-coloured sound-absorbent curtains and double glazing. Use comfortable ear plugs and eye shades.

- Make sure that your bedroom is well ventilated, and have some healthy indoor plants in your bedroom. The very green plants will make lots of oxygen to improve the air quality in your bedroom.
- Avoid sleeping in the daytime for more than one hour, or after 3 p.m.
- Try to go to bed by 10 p.m., as the body rests most efficiently between 10 p.m. and 6 a.m. This is a well-known and promoted habit for pilots, who need a high level of mental function. Try to be a creature of habit, at least during the week, and plan to go to bed at the same time every night.
- Try to avoid sleeping tablets, as they are addictive. Some cases of severe sleep disturbance are associated with a depressive illness, and in such cases anti-depressant drugs are much more effective at relieving insomnia, and are not nearly as addictive as sedatives or hypnotic drugs. Suitable anti-depressant drugs for relieving insomnia are the tricyclic drugs or the Selective Serotonin Re-uptake Inhibitors (SSRIs).
- Take regular exercise, as this produces an increase in the brain's endorphins, and improves circulation to the pineal gland.
- If you are overweight and have Syndrome X, follow the eating plan outlined on pages 115–22. This eating plan will lower your insulin levels and stabilize blood sugar levels, which will improve sleep apnoea (snoring) and breathing patterns during the night. Weight loss also reduces snoring.
- Talk to your doctor about using the natural hormone melatonin to improve your sleep.

# Chapter 15

# How Can I Reduce the Pain of Fibromyalgia?

As women get older and their production of hormones declines, the incidence of fibromyalgia increases.

Fibromyalgia is a common condition and describes the generalized aches and pains in the muscles, tendons, connective tissues and bones. There may be unpleasant sensations of stiffness and burning in the affected areas. The most common sites for fibromyalgic pain are the neck, shoulders, back and limbs. Fibromyalgia may be associated with:

- Auto-immune disease such as Lupus and rheumatoid arthritis
- Osteoporosis
- Periodontal disease (gum disease leading to loss of bone in the jaws and tooth loss)
- Headaches and chronic fatigue syndrome

### What Are the Causes?

Fibromyalgia is caused by:

- A decreasing production of the steroid hormones from the ovaries, and possibly the adrenal glands. The most important hormonal imbalances that can contribute to fibromyalgia involve the hormones oestrogen, DHEA, testosterone and pregnenolone.

- Mineral deficiencies will increase fibromyalgia and are very common in peri-menopausal women.
- Immune dysfunction with increasing inflammation in the connective tissues and bones
- Hidden infections in the body – these may be sub-clinical (not apparent) and may exist in the sinuses, respiratory tract, teeth, abdomen or pelvis and other parts of the body. These hidden infections release toxins which cause inflammation in the connective tissues. Chronic inflammation can show up by finding elevated levels of the protein globulins in the blood.
- A build-up of toxins and acidic waste products in the connective tissues and muscles, which cause pain, stiffness and tenderness

### How Can You Reduce Fibromyalgia?

- Regular exercise is vital – yoga, swimming, stretching, weight-bearing exercise and walking
- Some regular exposure to the sun can help to reduce pain; this is thought to be due to the increased production of vitamin D in the body, as well as a beneficial effect upon the immune system. Sun exposure is quite safe, provided you do not stay in the sun for more than 30 to 60 minutes at a time, and avoid direct exposure to the sun between the hours of 10 a.m. and 3 p.m., unless it is during the winter months. Many women avoid all exposure to the sun, and this has resulted in an increased incidence of vitamin D deficiency.
- Therapeutic massage, osteopathic treatments, physiotherapy and aromatherapy
- Drinking plenty of pure water
- Raw juicing is vital to overcome fibromyalgia – the best

vegetables and fruits to juice are celery, carrot, beetroot, apples, cabbage, watermelon and broccoli. Citrus juices can also help and can be mixed with apple and celery. Vitamin C in the citrus juices is a powerful anti-inflammatory agent. These juices should be drunk daily. They increase the elimination of toxic chemicals and reduce inflammation. If you add very small amounts of vegetables from the onion family (garlic, red onion, leeks and shallots), and horseradish and ginger root, the juice will exert a natural antibiotic effect, which can be effective in controlling hidden infections.

- Mineral supplementation is vitally important, as specific minerals are able to increase bone density and reduce inflammation.

The most important minerals to take are:
- calcium hydroxyapatite
- magnesium
- manganese
- zinc
- copper
- silica
- selenium

## OTHER SUPPLEMENTS THAT MAY REDUCE PAIN
- Vitamins D, C and E
- Glucosamine sulphate, which helps the joints and cartilage
- Organic sulphur in the form of Methyl-Sulphonyl-Methane (MSM)
  These are often available combined together in capsule or powder form.

## HRT for Fibromyalgia
Many women (and men) will find that their fibromyalgic pain

responds well to the use of natural HRT. The most important hormones for reducing pain and inflammation are:

- oestrogen and natural progesterone in women
- pregnenolone
- DHEA (Dehydroepiandrosterone)
- testosterone

It is not surprising that these hormones can exert anti-inflammatory and pain-relieving effects, as well as rejuvenating effects. This is because these hormones are all steroid hormones, and are therefore related in structure to natural cortisone, which is the most powerful anti-inflammatory hormone made in the human body.

Some sufferers of fibromyalgia experience a dramatic relief of their pain and tenderness after starting some of these hormones. Some patients will need to use all the mentioned hormones, which can easily be combined together into one cream or troche (lozenge).

Sometimes doctors prescribe a combination of creams and troches in one patient, to relieve fibromyalgia and menopausal symptoms. For example, in a woman with fibromyalgia, one could use the following daily regime: a troche containing a mixture of pregnenolone (50 to 100 mg), testosterone (2 to 10 mg) and DHEA (5 to 25 mg) plus a cream containing a mixture of oestradiol (0.5 to 2 mg) and progesterone (20 to 50 mg).

You can see that the range of possible therapeutic doses is quite large, and often in the long term, once the pain is under control, we will need to continue with only small doses. It is necessary to experiment with the doses of hormones initially, until one finds the most therapeutic doses and combinations.

**Case History**

I remember a patient who came to see me complaining of chronic pain in her back and neck. She had tried all types of anti-inflammatory drugs and pain killers, with no lasting relief. Her blood tests revealed very low levels of male hormones (androgens), as well as low oestrogen levels. She had undergone a hysterectomy 10 years before, after which her ovaries quickly stopped working.

Her chronic pain had started within six months of the hysterectomy, and although X-rays had shown some arthritis in the spine, it was not severe enough to account for all her pain.

I gave this woman an injection containing natural oestrogen and testosterone, and she came to see me one week later. She was very happy; her chronic aches and pains had completely gone and she felt energized and well. After six weeks the effect of the injection had worn off, however, and her pain returned. To keep her stable and relatively pain-free, I prescribed a troche containing a mixture of natural oestradiol 1 mg and testosterone 5 mg daily. She remains active, healthy and pain free; thankfully she no longer has to rely on pain killers and anti-inflammatory drugs. Without the troches, however, she finds that the pain returns, so she maintains taking these regularly. She also finds that she needs to take her mineral supplements regularly to keep the pain under control.

# Chapter 16

# Premature Menopause

Premature menopause is defined as ovarian failure occurring under the age of 40.

Spontaneous premature menopause occurs in approximately 1 per cent of women. There is an increased incidence of up to 10 per cent of premature menopause after gynaecological surgery or chemotherapy and/or radiotherapy for cancer.

## What Are Possible Causes of Premature Menopause?

- Chronic stress may upset the pituitary gland and thus the hormonal control of the ovaries.
- Auto-immune diseases may be associated with multiple gland failures, such as thyroid and adrenal dysfunction, as well as ovarian failure.
- Heavy smoking may damage the blood supply to the ovaries.
- Genetic factors – X chromosome deletions, or rare karyotypes such as 47XXX – can play their part.
- After gynaecological surgery – such as hysterectomy or removal of the ovaries.
- Chemotherapy and/or radiotherapy for cancer.

In many cases, however, the cause is unknown, and is due to what is called spontaneous premature ovarian failure.

### How Is Premature Menopause Diagnosed?

- There must be at least four months without menstrual bleeding.
- There must be elevated blood levels of the pituitary gland hormone called Follicle Stimulating Hormone (FSH), on two separate occasions, with the blood being tested for FSH levels at least 6 weeks apart. The FSH levels should be over 40mU/mL.

Other tests to help with a diagnosis include:

- oestrogen and progesterone blood levels, which would be low
- a trans-vaginal ultrasound scan to look for the existence of ovarian eggs (follicles)
- a DEXA Bone Density Test to check for osteoporosis
- chromosomal testing to check for genetic causes

Tests can also be done to exclude other causes of absent menstruation, which may **NOT** be due to premature ovarian failure. For example, other causes of absent or infrequent menstruation are:

- pregnancy
- extremes in body weight, especially very low body weight
- extreme exercise or sportive activity
- eating disorders, such as anorexia and/or bulimia
- drug addiction
- pituitary tumours producing high levels of the hormone prolactin
- ovarian tumours
- polycystic ovarian syndrome (PCOS) causing infrequent ovulation

- obstruction of blood flow in the uterus, cervix or vagina
- thyroid gland problems

## What Are the Symptoms of Premature Menopause?

The symptoms of premature menopause vary quite a lot depending upon if the failure of the ovaries occurs gradually or very suddenly.

This is why blood tests for FSH levels are so important, as they provide the definitive diagnosis.

### POSSIBLE SYMPTOMS
- absent menstruation
- loss of fertility
- irregular and/or infrequent periods
- very light or heavy periods
- mood disorders
- loss of libido
- vaginal dryness and discomfort during sex
- aches and pains
- night sweats and/or poor sleep
- fatigue

After surgical removal of the ovaries, or destruction of the ovaries by radiotherapy or chemotherapy, the onset of menopausal symptoms is usually sudden and often quite dramatic, especially in younger women.

### PROBLEMS ASSOCIATED WITH PREMATURE MENOPAUSE
- increased rate of bone loss
- possible increased risk of cardiovascular disease
- possible psychological, sexual and emotional problems
- premature loss of fertility – although in a significant percentage of women with premature ovarian failure the ovaries

may temporarily come back to life, and in around 10 per cent of cases a spontaneous pregnancy may subsequently occur. In women with true premature ovarian failure, we usually cannot get the ovaries to produce eggs that will ovulate. If these women wish to have children, they will need to consider adoption or receiving an ovarian egg from a donor.

## Psychological Issues of Premature Menopause

It is not uncommon for women with premature menopause, to experience a range of negative feelings such as:
- shock and disbelief
- a sense of great loss
- a sense of isolation from women of their own age group
- a sense of being cheated, especially if fertility is desired
- a sense of being different or abnormal
- a fear of premature ageing
- a fear of loss of sexuality

It is very important that, after the diagnosis is made, a woman has ample time and opportunity to express her emotions. Her partner, if she has one, should also be present for some discussion of the meaning of premature menopause. Some women erroneously believe that they have a disease, or that their relationships will never be the same; thus a lot of reassurance and positive feedback are required.

The term 'premature menopause' may conjure up negative connotations of being old, undesirable, barren or inadequate. It is more acceptable to the patient and her partner, family and friends to use the expression 'premature ovarian failure'.

Helpful web sites are www.whas.com.au and www.pofsupport.org

Treatment

The risk of osteoporosis is greater in women who have a premature menopause. In the past, relatively high-dose combined oral HRT or oral contraceptive pills have usually been prescribed. This has been done to relieve symptoms of oestrogen deficiency, and to preserve bone density. Indeed, many women have been or are given the oral contraceptive pill, as this induces a regular period, so that women will know they are not pregnant. This is comforting to women who feel that the 10 per cent spontaneous pregnancy rate after premature ovarian failure is unacceptable.

There are many types of HRT that can be prescribed. Generally a dose of oestrogen that is equivalent to 0.625 mg of Premarin or the 100-mcg oestrogen patches is used.

To produce a regular period (withdrawal bleed), a synthetic progestogen such as Provera is given for 12 to 14 days of each month.

Alternatively, micronized natural progesterone capsules in a dose of 100 to 200 mg can be used instead of synthetic progesterone. This type of treatment will help with symptoms of oestrogen deficiency, and may help well-being and sex drive; however, some women will also need testosterone. Testosterone can be given in the form of a cream, gel or troche (lozenge).

If the premature menopause was due to surgical removal of the uterus and/or ovaries, then many women find that implants of oestrogen and testosterone provide a complete relief of symptoms and greatly enhance their sex life. Natural progesterone can be given to balance these hormones, however it is not available in implants, so creams or troches will need to be prescribed.

The new-generation synthetic HRT called Livial (tibolone) can provide a welcome relief of symptoms, and also maintain bone density. Theoretically, Livial should be less likely to increase the incidence of breast cancer than conventional combined oral HRT, because Livial exerts an anti-oestrogenic effect upon the breast. I have had several patients who are taking Livial, who have told me that it has made a big improvement in the quality of their life. Other patients have told me that they have tried Livial and found that it made them feel 'bland' and caused weight gain. Once again this shows me that every woman's response to HRT is very individual.

In the light of the WHI study, which showed that long-term combined HRT using oral oestrogens and synthetic progestogens will increase the incidence of breast cancer and blood clots, a significant percentage of women with premature menopause will not feel comfortable about taking these tablets.

Thankfully we now have safer alternatives available for long-term HRT, such as hormone patches and creams; some women will also be candidates for oral natural oestrogens and natural progesterone.

Transdermal types of oestrogen (patches or creams) can be combined with a natural or synthetic progesterone and testosterone, if needed.

For a woman who loses her sex hormones under the age of 40, the prospect of a life without any sex hormones in her body can be daunting. She will probably live another 40 years, and she may feel totally sexless, tired and unfeminine. The use of natural therapies and mineral supplements can help greatly in the relief of symptoms and the maintenance of bone density; however when it comes to sexuality and sensuality, these natural therapies cannot replace the effect of real hormones. Thus most women with premature ovarian failure will want to try a combination of natural therapies and some form of HRT.

**Case History**

Jenny provides an interesting case history for younger women going through a premature ovarian failure. Jenny had undergone a hysterectomy when she was 38 years old, for severe endometriosis. Her disease had been so widespread that the surgeon had not been able to conserve her ovaries. Thus she had woken up from the operation with no uterus and no ovaries.

Within four days of the operation she had symptoms of severe hormone deficiency, and her hot flushes were so frequent that she was unable to sleep. Her gynaecologist had prescribed Trisequens tablets to be taken continuously, and these worked reasonably well for six months. Trisequens contains a combination of natural oestrogen and synthetic progesterone in one tablet.

Jenny had decided to see me because she had found that the hormone tablets she was taking had caused her to gain 12 kg (2 stone) in weight and had made her feel bloated. She also complained that, although she was now free of pelvic pain, she did not feel particularly feminine, and had no sex drive. Jenny had read about natural HRT, and wondered if it might suit her better.

Jenny's blood tests showed that she had reasonable levels of oestradiol, but very low levels of natural progesterone, and a very low free androgen index (FAI). This meant that, although she was receiving enough oestrogen, she was very deficient in natural progesterone and male hormones. The oral hormones that she was taking were making her liver produce excessive amounts of the hormone-binding protein called Sex Hormone Binding Globulin (SHBG). Her high levels of SHBG were binding the majority of the hormones in her bloodstream, which meant that her hormones were being inactivated.

I explained to Jenny that we needed to do several things to rebalance her hormones:

- reduce her high levels of SHBG, which would free up her active hormones
- increase her blood levels of natural progesterone
- increase her blood levels of natural testosterone
- maintain her blood oestrogen levels.

To achieve these changes, I recommended the following:

- that she stop the oral hormones, which could have been causing weight gain and bloating. The oral hormones were also increasing her SHBG levels.
- that she begin a troche (lozenge) containing a combination of Triest 2 mg, natural progesterone 40 mg and natural testosterone 1 mg daily, which she would place between the upper gum and the cheek until it was slowly absorbed through the cheek into the circulation.
- that she begin a hormone cream containing a mixture of oestradiol 1 mg, natural progesterone 20 mg and natural testosterone 1 mg, which she would massage into the vulva and clitoral area every night.
- that she start a raw juicing programme and take a liver tonic to promote weight loss and reduce fluid retention.

I asked her to return to see me after four months, at which stage I would retest her hormone levels.

After four months, Jenny's blood results showed that her hormones were now in the correct balance:

- Her progesterone levels were now in the normal range, and her SHBG had reduced considerably.
- Her FAI was back to normal levels.

Jenny told me that she was not surprised that her blood tests showed her hormones were back in balance. She had lost 8 kg (17½ pounds) and felt happy with her appearance. She was particularly happy about the improvement in her sex life; now she was free of pain and her hormones were back in balance, her sex life was better than it had been in many years, she said. She also felt much happier about the prospect of taking natural hormones long term than she had felt about taking synthetic progestogen.

# Chapter 17

# HRT – Should I Take It?

No matter what age a woman goes through the menopause, the question of whether to take any form of Hormone Replacement Therapy (HRT) remains an individual one. The length of time that a woman wants to stay on HRT is also a very individual decision, and is not a black-and-white matter. You will find that, as you age, your need for HRT and the doses of HRT that you require to alleviate symptoms may change greatly, and this is why you need to have a doctor with whom you can communicate well.

Since the results of the WHI study, the general consensus of opinion is not to use long-term oral HRT for the prevention of osteoporosis and/or cardiovascular disease. However, the fact that long-term HRT can reduce osteoporosis is well proven, and some women will decide, with their doctors, that they want to stay on HRT for the benefit of their bones. Of course, quality of life issues are very important too, and many women feel better mentally, physically and sexually on some form of HRT.

To help you to assess the relative benefits of HRT we can look at the profiles of two groups of women:

1. The profile of a higher-risk menopausal woman, who would generally do better with some form of HRT
2. The profile of a lower-risk menopausal woman, for whom HRT may not have as many benefits.

## Profile of a Higher-Risk Menopausal Woman

- premature menopause (age 40 or earlier)
- artificial menopause before the age of 45, caused by surgery, drugs, radiation or chemotherapy
- strong family history of cardiovascular disease
- sedentary lifestyle
- poor, nutrient-deficient diet
- sexual dysfunction and poor relationships
- depression and lack of enjoyment in life
- smoking
- fine build and small bone structure
- very low body weight
- low bone density, as determined from a DEXA bone scan

## Profile of a Lower-Risk Menopausal Woman

- menopause at age 50 (plus or minus 5 years)
- no family history of cardiovascular disease before the age of 65
- no family history of osteoporosis
- good bone density, as determined from a DEXA bone scan
- medium to heavy bone (skeletal) structure
- no history of depression
- a healthy nutrient rich diet
- non-smoker
- taking regular weight-bearing and aerobic exercise
- no long-term use of drugs that would increase bone loss (eg. steroids, excessively high doses of thyroid medication, some diuretics )

- a healthy cardiovascular system
- happy disposition and good relationships
- no problems with the sex life

Of course these hypothetical profiles fit women into well-defined categories, and this has limitations. This is a generalization and there will always be many exceptions to the rules. The most important thing to realize is that we can now cater for the women who are exceptions.

Since the results of the WHI study were published in August 2002, the opinion of the experts now stands divided between those who still recommend long-term HRT and those who do not. So the choice of whether you take HRT for long- or short-term use is no longer as clearly defined. It is now much more up to you and your own doctor to decide what is right for you!

I personally feel much more comfortable with this approach, as it involves *you* in the decision-making process to a much greater extent. It also takes us back to the good old days where the doctor worked more closely with the patient instead of being guided by the dictates of the drug companies.

The wonderful thing about modern-day HRT using natural bio-identical hormones is that we can now tailor-make a programme of HRT that takes into account all the individual characteristics and idiosyncrasies of each woman. This takes us way beyond the limitations, and greatly reduces the dangers, of using standard HRT protocols of synthetic hormones.

# Chapter 18

# Nutritional and Herbal Medicine for the Menopause

## Phytoestrogens

Phytoestrogens are substances found in plants that are converted into oestrogen-like compounds in the intestinal tract. Phytoestrogens found naturally in some plants, are structurally and functionally similar to human oestrogen, or produce oestrogen-like effects. Phytoestrogens can act on oestrogen receptors on the cell membranes, and have a balancing effect on oestrogen activity in the body. This balancing effect is called modulation, which sounds rather technical. What this means is that phytoestrogens can act to increase oestrogenic activity in the body when the body's own supply of oestrogen is too low, such as during the post-menopause. Conversely if the body's own natural oestrogen is too high, such as in oestrogen dominance, the phytoestrogens will reduce oestrogenic activity in the body.

Population studies have shown that consumption of a diet rich in phytoestrogens reduces oestrogen deficiency symptoms, and is protective against many types of cancer such as bowel, prostate, and breast cancer. A phytoestrogen rich diet also reduces the risk of cardiovascular disease and osteoporosis. Chinese and Japanese women have a lower reported incidence of menopausal symptoms, which is partly attributable to their phytoestrogen-rich diet.

## DIFFERENT TYPES OF PHYTOESTROGENS

- Isoflavones: there are 4 different isoflavones – genistein, biochanin, daidzein, and formononetin
- Lignans: These are converted to substances with biological oestrogenic effects
- Coumestans: Coumestrol is the collective name for the 20 coumestans that have been identified, and is the most potent of the phytoestrogens. It may be 30 to 100 times more active as an oestrogen than isoflavones, although theoretically 200 times less potent than the natural human hormone called oestrone.

## SOURCES OF PHYTOESTROGENS

| PHYTOESTROGEN | MAJOR SOURCE |
|---|---|
| Isoflavones | Soy and other beans, chickpeas, peas, fruits, spinach and other green vegetables, nuts, lentils, clovers, liquorice, sage, hops and some alcoholic drinks |
| Lignans | Seeds (especially **whole** flaxseed), nuts, cereals, spices, whole legumes, whole grains, fruits and vegetables, and dried seaweeds |
| Coumestans | Liquorice, peas, spinach, cabbage, soy bean sprouts, alfalfa sprouts, soy beans, green beans, mung beans and red clover |

Over 300 plants contain various combinations of phytoestrogens. These plant hormones are vital for the reproduction and defence-mechanisms of plants. Plant hormones are much weaker than human hormones, or hormones found in HRT.

Given their lack of potency, phytoestrogens are far less likely to cause hormonal imbalances in humans than are the synthetic hormones sometimes added to poultry and beef.

The table below compares the relative potency of different oestrogens. It is taken from *The Journal of Food Protection* (vol 42, 1979, pages 577–83).

| TYPE OF OESTROGEN | RELATIVE POTENCIES |
| --- | --- |
| Diethylstilboestrol (synthetic oestrogen) | 100,000.00 |
| Oestrogen (natural human) | 6,900.00 |
| Genistein (from soy) | 1.00 |
| Daidzein (from soy) | 0.75 |

**Note:** From the diagram on page 69, you can see the similarities in the chemical structure of oestradiol and an isoflavone compound. This similarity enables both molecules to bind to oestrogen receptors in the body.

## HEALTH BENEFITS OF ISOFLAVONES AND LIGNANS
- antioxidant action
- reduction of osteoporosis
- reduction of heart disease
- reduction of menopausal symptoms
- reduction of cancer

Plants containing phytoestrogens are on the list of cancer-preventative foods that have been studied within the USA Designer Food Program. This includes licorice, soy beans, flaxseed, barley and vegetables from the Brassicaceae family (cabbage, broccoli, Brussels sprouts, and cauliflower) and Umbelliferae (celery) family. The regular ingestion of plants from these families is strongly associated with a reduction in cancers of the breast, colon and lung, as well as other cancers.

## ARE SOY PRODUCTS BENEFICIAL?

Over the last several years there has been negative media coverage of soy beans and their products, such as tofu and tempeh. Much of the criticism is based on out-of-date information, and the detractors of soy have ignored many positive studies showing its beneficial health effects. Thousands of scientific studies have been published on soy and its derivatives; if you wish to do your own research you could begin by visiting the Medline database at *www.ncbi.nlm.nih.gov/PubMed/*.

Some of the critics of soy have said that it is more prone to cause allergic reactions. Soy is not especially toxic nor irritating to humans, as any food may cause allergies, and in this day and age all foods contain some naturally-occurring and introduced toxins.

Some of the critics of soy have warned women not to use any soy products in order to reduce the risk of hormone-dependent cancers, such as breast cancer. This logic is flawed and unsubstantiated.

The truth is that women (and men) should eat soy and other beans that are high in phytoestrogens, to reduce their risk of cancer. There are many good scientific articles that confirm that a diet high in soy, and other plants rich in isoflavones, reduce the incidence of hormone-dependent cancers such as breast and prostate cancer.

Many dietary surveys support a positive role in health for soy and its derivatives. Several studies, which measured the intake of phytoestrogens by urine tests, confirmed a significant reduction in the risk of breast cancer in women with a high intake of phytoestrogens.

Research has also shown that soy and its products contain several cancer-preventing substances such as genistein, saponins, carotenoids, trypsin inhibitors, phytates and flavonoids.

Critics have proclaimed that, '100 grams of soy protein can contain almost 600 mg of isoflavones, an amount that is undeniably toxic.' However, the critics should have given instances of harm in human beings caused by this amount of isoflavones. On average, 100 grams of soy protein contain 138 mg of isoflavones. Most soy recipes and meals contain around half a cup of soy per serving, which provides about 35 mg of isoflavones. The critics' comments pale into insignificance in the context of over 2,000 scientific articles on isoflavones, with the vast majority finding that isoflavones are very beneficial to health.

Populations ingesting diets high in legumes demonstrate significant health benefits, in particular a lower incidence of diseases that are epidemic in Western societies – namely bone diseases, cardiovascular disease and cancer. Dietary factors play a huge role in the genesis of these degenerative diseases, and the intake of dietary isoflavones is an important factor in reducing them. In East Asian diets, soy products such as tempeh, tofu and miso are the main sources of isoflavones. The traditional East Asian diet contains 20–60 mg of isoflavones daily, which is at least 10 times that of the modern Western diet, which contains only 2 to 5 mg.

Asian populations consuming a soy-rich diet have fewer bone fractures, fewer menopausal symptoms and fewer hormone-sensitive cancers than Western populations. Statistical analysis of food consumption among different populations provides definitive evidence for the protective effects of a diet high in soy and its derivatives.

Soy contains about 10 times more isoflavones than any other bean. The isoflavones in soy act to balance oestrogen in the body; specifically they are hormone-modulators, which mean they can down- or up-regulate body hormone receptors, as required.

Soy by itself is not a perfect protein; you must add two of the following food groups to soy, or indeed any legume, before it becomes a first-class protein:

- grains
- nuts
- seeds.

## Beneficial Effects of Soy Isoflavones

- reduce hormonal imbalances
- reduce menopausal symptoms
- lower cholesterol and triglycerides
- help to prevent osteoporosis
- reduce hormone dependent cancers.

## Increasing Your Dietary Intake of Phytoestrogens

- Drink herbal teas such as Alfalfa (Medicago) and Red Clover (Trifolium), two to three cups daily, sweetened with a little honey or stevia if desired. Alfalfa contains the phytoestrogen called coumestrol; red clover contains several isoflavones. Some women find that teas made from sage and hops also provide a welcome relief of symptoms.
- Eat 10 to 20 g of *whole* flaxseed daily – you can grind the seeds into a fine powder and sprinkle this on cereals or desserts, or add it to smoothies. It has a delicious sweet nutty taste! Alternatively you can soak the whole flaxseeds in water overnight and add them to breakfast cereal. Whole flaxseeds are very high in the phytoestrogens called lignans. You can also obtain additional lignans from wholegrains products.
- Replace some dairy products with soy products such as soy milk, soy cheese, soy yogurt and soy ice cream. Use soy beans, tempeh, tofu, miso and soy sauce in your recipes. Other beans also contain good amounts of valuable phytoestrogens.
- Include in your salads cooked beans of different varieties, cooked chickpeas, and raw seeds and alfalfa sprouts, which are high in phytoestrogens.

Herbal supplements and/or foods containing phytoestrogens can help with premenstrual syndrome, breast tenderness, endometriosis, heavy bleeding, menopausal symptoms and hair loss. The most effective herbs are:

- red clover
- wild yam
- black cohosh
- hops
- kelp
- alfalfa

You can obtain these herbs individually, or combined together in one formula called Femme Phase.

### PHYTOESTROGENS AND HRT

Phytoestrogens can still be used with great health benefits by women who are taking HRT. The phytoestrogens will help to complement the activity of the HRT upon the skin, hair, circulation and the bones. Remember that phytoestrogens also reduce your risk of many different types of cancer, so it is always wise to include them in your diet.

## Nutritional Medicine for the Menopause

The major health problems for women over 50 are:

- Osteoporosis
- A higher risk of cancer
- Cardiovascular diseases such as heart attacks and strokes
- The risk of degenerative diseases such as Alzheimer's disease and arthritis
- Depression and emotional problems
- Excessive weight gain and Type 2 diabetes

It is important that women utilize *preventative strategies* to reduce the occurrence of these common diseases. To keep these problems in check, some simple yet very powerful, dietary strategies can be followed.

I recommend the following:
- Drink at least 8 glasses of filtered, or rain water, every day.
- Start raw juicing – buy a juicer and drink fresh juices made from raw vegetables and fruits to increase your intake of antioxidants. There are many books on the market with detailed descriptions of raw juice recipes for many different problems, such as my book *Raw Juices can save your Life – The A–Z Guide of Juicing.*
- Use a grinder or food processor to grind fresh raw nuts and seeds such as flaxseeds, sesame seeds, sunflower seeds, pumpkin seeds and almonds, to provide essential fatty acids, fibre and minerals.
- Ensure an adequate intake of protein; good sources of protein are all seafood, organic eggs, organic chicken, lean red and white meats, legumes, whole grains, nuts and seeds, and whey protein powder. Some cheeses are also good sources of protein; the best cheeses for weight-watchers are parmesan, feta, cottage and ricotta cheeses. Ensure that you eat regular protein, as this will help you control your weight and reduce sugar cravings. It is also essential for those with the common metabolic disturbance of Syndrome X (see page 112). If you are vegan, you will need to be especially careful with food combining to ensure that you obtain first-class protein that contains all the essential amino acids required by the body. The basic rule to remember for obtaining first-class protein is that you need to combine *three* of the following four food groups at any one meal:

1. legumes (beans, peas and lentils)
2. nuts
3. seeds
4. grains

- Use **Super-Foods** – nutrient-dense foods that support the skeleton, nervous system, immune system and blood vessels – such as:

    Wheat grass juice
    Wheat germ (must be fresh)
    Lecithin (must be fresh)
    Garlic, leeks, shallots and red onions
    Citrus fruits
    Seaweeds such as arame, wakame, kombu, nori and kelp
    Alfalfa sprouts
    Legumes – beans, peas and lentils
    Cold-pressed seed and vegetable oils, especially flaxseed oil – this must be cold pressed and organic
    Tahini, hummus and natural nut spreads (instead of butter or margarine)
    Apple cider vinegar, which is a slimming aid and cleanser

- Follow **a regular exercise programme** that includes walking, swimming, recreational sports, light weight-training, yoga or tai chi. The exercise should include weight-bearing activities such as walking and/or using handweights. Handweights can be used while walking, moving in the swimming pool or dancing to some relaxing music. Yoga is very good at building muscle strength, improving co-ordination and relaxing the mind.

## SUPPLEMENTS

In all peri-menopausal and post-menopausal women, even those on HRT, nutritional supplements can be of great help in reducing osteoporosis and cardiovascular disease. They also help to slow down the ageing process, increase energy levels and improve memory.

The most useful supplements can be combined into what I call a 'Natural Menopause Kit':

- Essential fatty acids - from evening primrose oil, flaxseed oil, lecithin (available combined together in one capsule). Flaxseed oil can be used as a salad dressing, added to smoothies, poured on cereals or drunk from a spoon.
- Minerals to maintain and build healthy bones – the most efficient combination contains the minerals calcium hydroxyapatite and calcium citrate, magnesium, zinc, manganese, silica and copper
- Vitamins – E, D and C, which support the bones, blood vessels and the immune system
- Phytoestrogenic herbs available in the form of capsules or tinctures. An effective combination of herbs for menopausal symptoms is black cohosh, kelp, horsetail, wild yam, alfalfa, hops and red clover.
- Organic sulphur such as Methyl-Sulphonyl-Methane (MSM) can support liver function and is able to reduce hair loss and ageing of the skin.
- The mineral selenium (in the organic form of selenomethionine) is very important for the immune system. Selenium is able to reduce the risk of many types of cancer, and also reduces inflammation. Selenium is also vital for the efficient functioning of the thyroid gland. Selenium can be used as an effective anti-ageing tool.

No matter what age you are when you go through the menopause, you will have fewer symptoms and feel healthier if you have a good diet, a regular exercise program, a positive state of mind and a healthy liver. The liver breaks down (metabolizes) all the body's hormones, as well as any HRT that is being prescribed. If the liver is sluggish or dysfunctional, hormonal imbalances can arise. Peri-menopausal women with sluggish liver function are more likely to have a weight problem, because the liver is the major fat-burning organ in the body. Liver tonic powders such as Livatone can help to control weight excess.

The Menopause is a natural phase of your life, and it is not surprising that women are turning increasingly towards the most natural solutions for their symptoms. A healthy diet and the use of a phytoestrogen supplement can help to achieve these goals.

The aim of these natural approaches is to maintain a healthy balance of the body's hormones and to keep the immune system strong. A healthy immune system is your greatest health asset, and the liver is the protector of the immune system.

I recommend that you only purchase natural menopause products that contain a *standardized dose of isoflavones.* They may be slightly more expensive, but it is worth it because at least you know that you will be getting the proven benefits of a known dose of isoflavones. The isoflavones are the phytoestrogens that exert hormone-balancing and bone-preserving effects in women.

# Herbal Medicine and Natural Remedies for the Menopause

| HERB | BENEFITS |
|---|---|
| Black Cohosh (Cimicifuga racemosa) | May reduce hot flushes and period cramps. Helpful for reducing muscular pain and cramping. The active principle is saponins, which are not phytoestrogens. |
| Wild Yam (Dioscorea villosa) | Is a mild aphrodisiac and may increase sex drive. Exerts an anti-inflammatory effect, which may reduce arthritic pain. Wild yam contains the plant hormone called diosgenin, which is used commercially to manufacture natural progesterone and other prescription hormones. The diosgenin from wild yam is not converted in the body into human progesterone. |
| Hops (Humulus lupulus) | Is an oestrogenic herb that may reduce hot flushes, night sweats and vaginal dryness. This herb has a mild sedative effect, which is useful in anxiety and insomnia. The hormonal activity of hops has long been recognised, as women harvesting hops may experience menstrual changes. |
| Sage (medicago sativa) | This herb has many medicinal properties, and is useful for the relief of hot flushes and sweating. You can take sage as part of a menopause formula, or drink sage tea, slightly sweetened with honey, or stevia. You may sprinkle finely chopped sage on soups, salads and vegetables. |
| Red Clover (Trifolium pratense) | Red clover is a source of the isoflavones formononetin, daidzein, biochanin and genistein. |

| | |
|---|---|
| Red Clover (Trifolium pratense) cont. | These act as plant oestrogens known as phyto-estrogens. Red clover is useful for relieving hot flushes and may help bone density. |
| Dong Quai (Angelica polymorpha or sinensis) | May help to reduce hot flushes and improve fatigue, although some studies have found that it is no better than a placebo. Higher doses have been linked with breast lumps. |
| St Johns Wort (Hypericum perforatum) | Is specific for mild depression and anxiety. It must NOT be taken concurrently with anti-depressant drugs. |
| Damiana (Turnera Diffusa) | Traditionally has been used as a 'hormone balancer' and may help to reduce hot flushes. Can have aphrodisiac properties. High doses may cause urinary irritation. |
| Dandelion (Taraxacum Officinale) and St Mary's Thistle (Silybum Marianum) | These herbs act on the liver to improve its function, and may repair liver damage. Some women find that these herbs greatly reduce hot flushes. They help with weight loss and detoxification. |
| Liquorice (Glycyrrhiza Glabra) contains several different isoflavones | Exerts oestrogenic effects. Liquorice is an adrenal tonic, and may help with dizziness, low blood pressure, hypoglycaemia and fatigue. Very high doses may elevate the blood pressure slightly, deplete potassium and cause fluid retention, although I have never had any problems with liquorice in my patients. It can be used as part of a menopausal formula, and also drunk as a pleasant tasting herbal tea. |

| | |
|---|---|
| Chaste tree (Vitex-agnus castus) | Has been used traditionally to help women with a progesterone deficiency, although there is no clinical proof of this. Some women find it helpful for Premenstrual Syndrome. |
| Kelp (Fucus vesiculosis) | Is an excellent source of many minerals, including iodine. Helpful for an under active thyroid gland and hair loss. |
| Horsetail (Equisetum arvense) | This herb is high in the mineral silica, which increases bone strength and improves the nails and the strength of the hair shaft. |
| Horsechestnut | Is beneficial for the blood vessels, and is of benefit for varicose veins and broken capillaries. |
| Sarsaparilla (Smilas Officinalis) | Has been used traditionally as a tonic, and has mild aphrodisiac properties. |
| Ginseng | The different types of Ginseng do not contain phytoestrogens. Ginseng may help reduce menopausal fatigue and stress because it has a tonic effect upon the adrenal glands. |
| Flaxseed (linseed) The whole seed comprising the fibrous parts are high in the phytoestrogenic lignans. The oil is not high in phytoestrogens but contains valuable essential fatty acids. | Is a good source of the phytoestrogens called lignans, which reduce menopausal symptoms. Reduces dryness of the vagina and skin. Can reduce cholesterol levels and reduce cardiovascular disease. Improves the appearance of the skin and hair. |

| Cruciferous vegetables (cabbage, broccoli, cauliflower, Brussels sprouts) | These contain the substance called indole-3-carbinol, which is considered to be a phyto-estrogen by many researchers. This may help the liver detoxification pathways that break down oestrogen. Diets high in cruciferous vegetables reduce the risk of many types of cancer. |
| --- | --- |

# Chapter 19

# Relief of Menopausal Symptoms

| SYMPTOMS | MEDICATION | NATURAL REMEDY |
|---|---|---|
| Hot flushes | Oestrogen in the form of creams, gels, patches, sprays, troches, implants, injections and tablets.<br>Livial tablets. | Improve liver function with raw vegetable juices and liver tonic capsules or powder. Hot flushes and sweating can be due to a dysfunctional or fatty liver.<br>Weight loss can help reduce hot flushes.<br>The herbs red clover, black cohosh, hops, sage and peppermint.<br>Alfalfa sprouts and soybeans. |
| Dryness and discomfort in the vagina.<br>Bladder and urinary problems | Oestrogen in the form of vaginal cream or vaginal pessaries, or the vaginal ring called ESTring. | Cold pressed flaxseed oil and evening primrose oil.<br>Natural vitamin E.<br>Selenium.<br>Raw vegetable juicing.<br>The herbs golden seal, sage, hops and marshmallow. |

| | | |
|---|---|---|
| Poor memory and reduced mental function | Pregnenolone and oestrogen in the form of troches or creams. | Cold pressed flaxseed oil. Lecithin. Vitamin B complex. Vitamin C. Raw vegetable juicing to provide folic acid, which reduces the risk of dementia. The herbs Ginkgo Biloba and Bilberry, which improve circulation to the brain. |
| Poor sleep and anxiety | Oestrogen and natural progesterone in the form of creams, patches or troches. | Magnesium Complete. Regular protein meals. The herbs valerian and hops. |
| Depression | Oestrogen and natural progesterone. Natural testosterone and DHEA. In severe cases a SSRI anti-depressant drug may work very well. | St John's Wort (hypericum). Magnesium Complete. Cold pressed flaxseed oil. Vitamin C. Vitamin B complex. |
| Fibromyalgia | Pregnenolone, DHEA and natural testosterone in creams and troches. Natural oestrogen and progesterone can also reduce inflammation. Anti-inflammatory drugs and/or analgesics (containing paracetamol | Raw juicing. Vitamin D and some gentle sun baking. Mineral supplements containing – Calcium hydroxyapatite, selenium, magnesium, zinc, manganese, copper and silica. Glucosamine sulphate. The herbs horsetail, yucca, or white willow bark. Massage and exercise. |

| | | |
|---|---|---|
| | and codeine) can be used for acute attacks. | |
| Hair loss | Natural progesterone in creams or troches. Avoid testosterone. If excess male hormones are present in a blood test (elevated Free Androgen Index – FAI), the hormone cyproterone acetate may help greatly. | MSM and Vitamin C powder. Flaxseed oil. The herbs horsetail and kelp, which provide silica and other minerals. Selenium and zinc. Phytoestrogens see pages 210–11 If weight excess in the upper body and abdomen is present, weight loss will help to reduce hair loss. |
| Wrinkling of the skin | Oestrogen and natural progesterone and DHEA in the form of creams or troches. | Avoid smoking and excess alcohol, as these accelerate ageing of the skin. Natural Vitamin E. Selenium and zinc. MSM and Vitamin C powder. Raw juicing. Cold pressed flaxseed oil. |
| Sexual problems and poor libido | Oestrogen, testosterone and/or DHEA in the form of implants, injections, creams or troches. | The herbs Wild yam, Tribulus and Horny goat weed. |
| Weight gain | Avoid synthetic hormone tablets, and use creams or patches containing natural hormones. | Follow the Syndrome X Eating Plan in chapter 23 of the book titled *Can't Lose Weight? You could have Syndrome X* |

| Weight gain *cont.* | Avoid testosterone and use DHEA instead. The drug Xenical reduces the absorption of fat from the gut after a meal, but may cause digestive problems. The drug Reductil reduces the appetite and must be prescribed by a doctor. These drugs have a useful role in severe obesity. | Take a liver tonic capsule such as Livatone to help the liver burn fat. Raw vegetable juicing to improve the liver function. Synd-X Slimming Protein Powder to ensure regular protein intake. The herbs Brindle Berry, Bitter Melon and Gymnema Sylvestre improve the metabolism. The mineral chromium picolinate reduces cravings. For more information see www.weightcontroldoctor.com |
|---|---|---|
| Osteoporosis | Natural oestrogen, progesterone and testosterone can reduce bone loss. Evista (Raloxifene) tablets reduce bone loss. Rocaltrol and the Bisphosphonate drugs, such as Alendronate (Fosamax), can build bone. | A mineral supplement such as a complete calcium formula combining – <br>• Calcium hydroxyapatite<br>• Calcium citrate<br>• Magnesium<br>• Manganese<br>• Zinc<br>• Copper<br>• Vitamin D<br>Regular weight-bearing exercises are essential. Avoid smoking. |

# Chapter 20

## Prescription Hormones – Natural and Synthetic

### Prescription Hormones and Their Effects

| HORMONE TYPE | BENEFITS | DAILY DOSES | POSSIBLE SIDE-EFFECTS | SOLUTION TO SIDE-EFFECTS |
|---|---|---|---|---|
| **Natural Human Oestrogens** <br> • Oestradiol <br> • Oestriol <br> • Oestrone <br><br> **Equine Oestrogens** such as Premarin <br><br> **Synthetic Oestrogens** such as Ethynyl-oestradiol <br><br> Oestrogens are avail-able in the form of – <br> • Tablets <br> • Implants <br> • Patches <br> • Injections <br> • Lozenges (troches) | Reduce acne and facial hair. Improve skin texture. Improve vaginal lubrication. Increase size of vaginal lips (vulva) and clitoris. Increase the sensitivity of the clitoris. Reduce bladder control prob-lems. Increase the sex drive. Improve the ability to orgasm. Prevent shrinkage of the vagina. May increase breast size. Increase sensitivity of the nipples. Improve sleep and reduce hot flushes. Reduce loss of bone density. May reduce depression and improve mental function. | 0.5 mg to 4 mg. These doses can vary great-ly, according to the patient's needs. | Increased risk of blood clots. Aggravation of liver - gall bladder problems. Nausea. Increased risk of strokes. Increase in blood pressure. Leg cramps and aching legs. Aggravation of varicose veins. Weight gain. Migraines. Fluid retention. Abdominal bloating and cramps. Period pains. Breast tenderness and swelling. Long term use of high doses will increase the risk of breast cancer. Break-through bleeding. Increase in the amount of menstrual bleeding. | If side-effects are severe, the oestrogen must be stopped. However, generally speaking, oestrogenic side-effects can be reduced or eliminated by <br> • Reducing the dose of oestrogen – often only very small doses will be required. <br> • Using a more natural oestrogen <br> • Using the weaker oestrogen, called oestriol <br> • Giving oestrogen in the form of a cream or patch |

| HORMONE TYPE | BENEFITS | DAILY DOSES | POSSIBLE SIDE-EFFECTS | SOLUTION TO SIDE-EFFECTS |
|---|---|---|---|---|
| • Creams<br>• Vaginal rings<br>• Gels<br>• Nasal sprays<br>may soon be available | May improve cholesterol levels.<br>Oestrogen often reduces aches and pains and the symptoms of fibromyalgia. | | Increase in the size of uterine fibroids.<br>Increase in the thickness of the uterine lining (endometrial hyperplasia). | • Using oestrogen cream in the vaginal area only |
| **New Generation Hormones**<br><br>These are synthetic and are known as **Estro-progestins** – an example of these drugs is Livial (Tibolone).<br>Livial exerts oestrogenic effects, progestogenic effects and andro-genic effects. Thus | Reduce vaginal dryness and atrophy. May improve the sex life.<br>Reduce hot flushes and sweats.<br>Reduce bone loss.<br>Livial has anti-oestrogenic and progesto-genic effects on the breast.<br>Is said not to stimulate the uterus, therefore bleeding does not occur as often as it does with conventional HRT. | One 2.5 mg tablet daily | May decrease the levels of the good HDL cholesterol, which may have an adverse effect upon cardiovascular disease.<br>Weight gain.<br>Aggravation of liver disease.<br>Increased risk of blood clots.<br>Elevation of blood pressure.<br>Abdominal swelling and cramps.<br>Breast pain.<br>Possible increased risk of breast cancer. | Cease the medication.<br>If side-effects occur, more natural types of HRT in low doses will be more acceptable. |

| HORMONE TYPE | BENEFITS | DAILY DOSES | POSSIBLE SIDE-EFFECTS | SOLUTION TO SIDE-EFFECTS |
|---|---|---|---|---|
| Livial, although it is **one** hormone, acts like 3 different hormones, having female and male hormone effects.<br><br>Estro-progestins are available as tablets. | | | | |
| **New Generation Hormones**<br>These are synthetic and are known as **Selective Estrogen Receptor Modulators = (SERMs)**<br>eg. Evista (Raloxifene)<br>The action of this | The SERM drugs are predominantly used to prevent and treat osteoporosis in post-menopausal women.<br>They may have a beneficial effect upon the blood fats such as reducing the bad LDL cholesterol.<br>They do not stimulate the growth of the uterine lining, and thus do not produce periods. | One 60mg tablet daily | Increased risk of blood clots. Aches and cramps in the legs.<br>They do not reduce hot flushes, and indeed may increase them.<br>They may aggravate liver disease.<br>Weight gain and fluid retention.<br>Migraines.<br>Elevation of blood pressure. | Cease the medication. If side-effects occur, more natural types of HRT in low doses will be more acceptable. |

| HORMONE TYPE | BENEFITS | DAILY DOSES | POSSIBLE SIDE-EFFECTS | SOLUTION TO SIDE-EFFECTS |
|---|---|---|---|---|
| class of drugs is complicated and they act to stimulate some of the body's oestrogen receptors, and block some of the other oestrogen receptors. Thus they can exert both oestrogenic effects, and anti-oestrogenic effects on different oestrogen receptors, which exist on the body cells. For example, Raloxifene, appears to block the effect of oestrogen upon the breast and uterus. Many women will find this difficult to understand. They are available as tablets. | They do not seem to produce breast tenderness however the long term effect of Raloxifene upon the risk of breast cancer, is unknown. | | They do not help vaginal dryness or the sex life. | Cease the medication. If side-effects occur, more natural types of HRT, in lower doses will be more acceptable. |

| HORMONE TYPE | BENEFITS | DAILY DOSES | POSSIBLE SIDE-EFFECTS | SOLUTION TO SIDE-EFFECTS |
|---|---|---|---|---|
| **Natural Human Progesterone**<br>Available as –<br>• Creams<br>• Lozenges (troches)<br>• Capsules (the capsules contain micronised progesterone to increase absorption)<br>• Injections | Reduction in mood disorders such as anxiety and depression. Reduction in the amount of menstrual bleeding and reduced period pains.<br>Studies have shown that natural progesterone given vaginally may reduce endometrial hyperplasia in over 90% of women. Thus natural progesterone can reduce the risk of uterine cancer.<br>Reduction in the size of uterine fibroids, period pains and endometriosis.<br>May increase fertility and reduce early miscarriage rates. May overcome the majority of the symptoms of the Premenstrual Syndrome (PMS). Is extremely helpful for women with ovulation | Doses required vary greatly according to the reason that natural progesterone is being prescribed.<br>To reduce heavy bleeding and endometrial hyperplasia, doses of 100 mg daily are needed, and this is best given vaginally. For PMS doses can vary between 25 to 100 mg daily and this can be given in the form of creams or lozenges. Dr Katharina Dalton, who was a pioneer in the use of natural progesterone, often used large doses of natural progesterone of up to 400 mg daily.<br>If natural progesterone | If excess doses are used, women may complain of drowsiness and fatigue, headaches, abdominal cramps and bloating or constipation.<br>If excess amounts of vaginal cream are used, or if the cream contains irritants, then vaginal irritation may occur.<br>Fluid retention.<br>Weight gain. | Usually side-effects can be completely overcome by reducing the dose. Some women may find that the troches do not suit them, in which case, progesterone cream is usually better tolerated. |

| HORMONE TYPE | BENEFITS | DAILY DOSES | POSSIBLE SIDE-EFFECTS | SOLUTION TO SIDE-EFFECTS |
|---|---|---|---|---|
| | problems, such as Polycystic ovarian syndrome and peri-menopausal hormonal imbalances.<br>Improves wellbeing.<br>Improvement in the hair, with a reduction of hair loss.<br>Does not exert an adverse effect upon blood fats or glucose (sugar) metabolism.<br>May be helpful in women with multiple sclerosis and premenstrual epilepsy. | is being taken along with oestrogen to relieve symptoms of menopause, then we may need to use higher doses of progesterone if the woman still has her uterus. | | |
| Natural Human Testosterone<br>Available as creams, lozenges (troches), gels, patches or implants.<br>Testosterone tablets and injections are | Improves mood and reduces depression.<br>Increases energy and physical strength.<br>May reduce panic attacks.<br>Restores the libido and the ability to orgasm.<br>Increases the size and sensi- | Doses vary greatly from 0.2 mg to 5 mg daily in women, depending upon symptoms and the results of blood tests.<br>Men may need higher doses. | Side-effects are very dependent upon the doses used, and very small doses do not usually have significant side-effects.<br>Increase in facial and/or body hair. | Reduce the doses used.<br>Avoid synthetic testosterone.<br>Use the creams, or patches, as these are less likely to cause side-effects. |

| HORMONE TYPE | BENEFITS | DAILY DOSES | POSSIBLE SIDE-EFFECTS | SOLUTION TO SIDE-EFFECTS |
|---|---|---|---|---|
| also available, however they are often synthetic. Now that we have natural testosterone, there is no need to use synthetic or potent doses of testosterone in women. | tivity of the clitoris. Reduces aches and pains and fibromyalgia. Increases bone density. | | Increased hair loss from the scalp. Increase in pimples, acne and oily skin. Increase in the bad LDL cholesterol. Weight gain. Increased muscle mass. Enlargement of the prostate gland. | |
| Natural Dehydro-epiandrosterone (DHEA) Available in lozenges (troches), capsules and creams | Increases energy levels and well being. Increases libido. May improve depression and mood disorders. Reduces aches and pains and fibromyalgia. Can be useful in cases of adrenal gland exhaustion and chronic fatigue syndrome. May increase bone density. May have anti-ageing effects. | Doses vary from 2.5 to 25 mg daily in women, and 25 to 100 mg daily in men. | Acne and oily skin Facial and body hair Headaches Weight gain DHEA can stimulate the growth of tumour cells. Increase in size of the prostate gland. | Reduce dose of DHEA. Change to DHEA creams instead of oral forms. |

| HORMONE TYPE | BENEFITS | DAILY DOSES | POSSIBLE SIDE-EFFECTS | SOLUTION TO SIDE-EFFECTS |
|---|---|---|---|---|
| Natural Human Pregnenolone Available in lozenges (troches), capsules and creams | Pregnenolone is a natural steroid hormone, and as such may help to relieve the symptoms of a range of inflammatory disorders such as – <br>• Arthritis <br>• Fibromyalgia <br>• Auto-immune disorders such as Lupus, psoriasis and eczema <br>• Multiple sclerosis <br>Improves memory and mental performance. <br>Reduces the negative effects of stress. These beneficial effects can be very powerful. Can be useful in cases of adrenal gland dysfunction or exhaustion. <br>Pregnenolone is a much under rated hormone. It really should be used more often to help patients with the above problems. | Doses vary from 10 mg to 100 mg daily | Pregnenolone is generally free of side-effects. If excess doses are used, fluid retention or a mild agitation may occur. | Reduce the dosage or change to creams. |

| HORMONE TYPE | BENEFITS | DAILY DOSES | POSSIBLE SIDE-EFFECTS | SOLUTION TO SIDE-EFFECTS |
|---|---|---|---|---|
| **Synthetic Progesterones** are known as **Progestogens** Examples are Medroxy- progesterone acetate (brand names Provera and Ralovera), Norethisterone, and Dydrogesterone (Duphaston) | If given cyclically for 12 to 14 days of the month, the progestogens will produce a regular period. They reduce the amount of menstrual bleeding and pain. May reduce endometriosis and fibroids. Reduce the risk of uterine cancer. Generally they do not have androgenic (male hormone-like effects), although Norethisterone is more likely to cause masculine side-effects, than are the other progestogens. | Provera and Ralovera tablets 2.5, 5, 10, and 100 mg. Norethisterone tablets 2.5 to 5 mg. Dydrogesterone tablets 10 mg. | Progestogens are more potent than natural progesterone. They may cause fluid retention, weight gain and nausea. Impairment of glucose tolerance. Depression and PMS. Dizziness. Blood pressure elevation. Blood clots. Headaches. Sleep disturbances. Hair loss. | Reduce dosage of progestogen or change to a natural progesterone. Natural progesterone is far less likely to cause side-effects. |

| HORMONE TYPE | BENEFITS | DAILY DOSES | POSSIBLE SIDE-EFFECTS | SOLUTION TO SIDE-EFFECTS |
|---|---|---|---|---|
| **Anti-male Hormones** These are synthetic and block the action of the male hormones in the body. eg. Cyproterone acetate (Brand names Androcur, Cyprone and Procur) | Cyproterone acetate is a hormone with 2 actions. It is both an Anti-male hormone and Progestogen. It is very effective in treating the symptoms of excess male hormones. Cyproterone acetate can greatly reduce and control – Excess facial and body hair. Acne and greasy skin. Hair loss from the scalp due to androgen excess. Because of its progestogen effect, it can also reduce heavy bleeding and if given cyclically it can produce a regular menstrual bleed. Can reduce period pain. In women with excess male hormones (androgens), which are contributing to Syndrome X and weight excess, cyproterone may help with weight loss. | 2 to 100 mg tablets daily. | The side-effects are very much related to the dosage used. Cyproterone acetate may cause fatigue, depression, and a reduction in sex drive. It may cause fluid retention and headaches. | Side-effects can usually be overcome by reducing the dose to much lower levels. Some women only need very small amounts of cyproterone acetate to control their symptoms of excess male hormones. |

Here is a table that you may find helpful if you are taking conventional HRT and wish to switch to natural hormone creams.

| ORAL OESTROGENS | USUAL DAILY DOSE | EQUIVALENT DOSE OF TRIEST CREAM |
|---|---|---|
| **Ogen or Genoral** Contains piperazine oestrone sulphate | 0.625–1.25 mg | 2–4 mg |
| **Premarin** Contains conjugated equine (horse) and human oestrogens | 0.625–1.25 mg | 2–4 mg |
| **Progynova** Contains oestradiol valerate | 1–2 mg | 2–3 mg |
| **Zumenon or Estrofem** Contains micronised oestradiol hemi-hydrate | 1–2 mg | 2–3 mg |
| **OESTROGEN PATCHES** | | EQUIVALENT DOSE OF TRIEST CREAM |
| **Estraderm, Femtran, Menorest, Climara, Dermestril** These are all brand names of oestrogen patches | USUAL DOSE 25mcg/24hours 50mcg/24hours 75mcg/24hours 100mcg/24hours | 1 mg 2 mg 3 mg 4 mg |

This table may help if you are taking synthetic progesterone (progestogen) and wish to switch to natural progesterone capsules or troches.

| SYNTHETIC PROGESTOGEN | USUAL DOSE | EQUIVALENT DOSE OF NATURAL PROESTERONE |
|---|---|---|
| Provera or Ralovera<br>Contains medroxy-progesterone acetate | 2.5–10 mg | 50–200 mg |
| Duphaston<br>Contains dydrogesterone | 5–10 mg | 100–200 mg |
| Primolut<br>Contains norethisterone | 1 mg | 200 mg |

## Brands of Prescription Hormones for the Female Menopause

### OESTROGENS
#### Patches
Climara       Oestradiol in 25/50/75/100 – once weekly
Dermestril    Oestradiol in 25/50/100 – twice weekly
Estraderm     Oestradiol in 25/50/75/100 – twice weekly
Femtran       Oestradiol in 50/100 – once weekly
Menorest      Oestradiol in 37.5/50/75/100 – twice weekly
Estracombi    Oestradiol + Norethisterone acetate
Estalis       Oestradiol + Norethisterone acetate

**Tablets**

| | |
|---|---|
| Progynova | Oestradiol valerate 1- and 2- mg tablets |
| Zumenon | Oestradiol hemihydrate 2 mg |
| Estrofem | Oestradiol 1-, 2- and 4- mg tablets |
| Climen | Oestradiol valerate 2 mg + Androcur 1 mg |
| Divina | Oestradiol valerate 2 mg + Provera 10 mg |
| Kliovance | Oestradiol hemihydrate 1 mg + Norethis-terone 0.5 mg |
| Trisequens | Oestradiol 1, 2 and 4 mg + Norethis-terone acetate 1 mg |
| Femoston | Oestradiol 2 mg + Dydrogesterone 10 mg |
| Ovestin | Oestriol 1-mg tablet |
| Ogen | Oestrone piperazine sulfate 0.625 mg, 1.25 mg |
| Premarin | Mixture of equine oestrogens in doses of 0.3, 0.625 and 1.25 mg |
| Premia | Premarin 0.625 mg + Provera 5 mg |
| Provelle | Premarin 0.625 mg + Provera 10 mg |
| Menoprem | Premarin 0.625 mg + Provera 10 mg |

**Gels**

Sandrena Oestradiol in alcohol based gel 1 mg/gm gel in sachets.

**Creams**

The creams can be compounded to contain any combination and dose of the body's three natural oestrogens, namely oestradiol, oestriol and oestrone. Other hormones, such as progesterone, DHEA, pregnenolone and testosterone may be added if needed.

**Troches (Lozenges)**

The troches can be compounded to contain any combination and dose of the body's three natural oestrogens, namely oestradiol, oestriol and oestrone. Other hormones, such as progesterone, DHEA, pregnenolone and testosterone may be added in the same troche if needed.

## Implants

| | |
|---|---|
| Oestradiol hemihydrate | Oestradiol 20-, 50- or 100-mg implants |
| Testosterone | Testosterone 100- and 200-mg implants |
| Made by Organon | |

## Injections

| | |
|---|---|
| Primogyn Depot injection | Oestradiol valerate in oily base, 10mg ampoules |

## Nasal Spray

| | |
|---|---|
| Aerodiol | Oestradiol hemihydrate in a glass bottle/with metering pump. |

## Vaginal Ring

| | |
|---|---|
| EString | Oestradiol 2 mg. The ring is inserted into the upper part of the vagina. It is worn continuously for 3 months, and is then replaced with a new ring. |

## ANTI-MALE HORMONES

| | |
|---|---|
| Androcur tablets | Cyproterone acetate 50-mg tablets |
| Cyprone tablets | Cyproterone acetate 50-mg tablets |
| Procur tablets | Cyproterone acetate 50-mg tablets |

## NATURAL PROGESTERONE

| | |
|---|---|
| Proluton Depot Injection | Progesterone 25 mg, in oily base |
| Lozenges (troches) | Progesterone in a tailor-made dosage |
| Capsules | Progesterone in micronized form in tailor-made dose |

**Creams**

Progesterone in a tailor-made dosage

**Pessaries – vaginal**

Progesterone in a tailor-made dosage

**SYNTHETIC PROGESTERONE** (known as progestogen)

| | |
|---|---|
| Provera tablets | Medroxyprogesterone acetate 2.5-, 5- and 10-mg tablets |
| Ralovera tablets | Medroxyprogesterone acetate 2.5-, 5- and 10-mg tablets |
| Duphaston tablets | Dydrogesterone 10-mg tablets |
| Primolut tablets | Norethisterone 5-mg tablets |

**For the Male Menopause**

**TESTOSTERONE**

**Tablets**

| | |
|---|---|
| Andriol | Testosterone undecanoate 40 mg |
| Proviron | Mesterolone 25 mg |

**Patches**

| | |
|---|---|
| Androderm | Testosterone, dissolved in alcohol based gel – 2 patches provides testosterone 5 mg daily |

**Injections**

| | |
|---|---|
| Primoteston injection | Testosterone enanthate 250 mg in oily base |
| Sustanon injection | A mixture of testosterone propionate, phenylpropionate and isocaproate in 100- and 250-mg ampoules |

**Implants**

| | |
|---|---|
| Testosterone (Organon) | Testosterone 100- and 200-mg implants |

# Farewell

I sincerely hope that this book has helped to clear up some of the confusion surrounding the use of hormone replacement therapy for menopausal women. I have presented the facts as I find them, both in the literature and in my clinical practice. I have no partic-ular wheelbarrow to push and no vested interest in HRT, and thus I have presented an unbiased perspective on the use of hormone replacement therapy for all women. I personally use natural hor-mone replacement therapy, and I have found it produced a great improvement in my well-being and I certainly will not be giving it up! However I use only natural hormones, and would never take any synthetic hormones. I am sure for the thousands of women who wish to continue with some form of HRT, that this book will give them new guidance in their lives as they get older.

HRT will always remain a popular, emotive and controversial subject because –

- It is powerful stuff – it can change your life in a positive way.
- It is a sexual and incredibly sensual subject – yes it is true that hormones make the world go round!
- It is part of a woman's identity.

- It generates billions of dollars for drug companies.
- It polarizes and impassions researchers, academics and clinicians.
- It challenges doctors who are faced with the pressure of needy women and litigation.
- It generates millions of dollars for the media.
- It is part of anti-ageing medicine and the world supports an increasingly ageing population.

So controversial or not, hormone replacement therapy, in its many forms, will not become a thing of the past. Millions of words will continue to be spoken and written about hormone replacement therapy, as new research becomes available. There is an urgent need for ongoing research into the use of more natural types of hormones, to relieve symptoms and improve the quality of life for women.

Our level of understanding of hormones can only increase, which will benefit society, and especially women, who must continue to go through the menopause, until we can re-programme the genes that control the extinction of our ovarian eggs.

Way back in the 1930s, we began giving women natural replicas of their own hormones, and women jumped at this opportunity to replace the hormones they no longer produced. Drug companies then realized that there was more money to be made in creating artificial hormones, or using cross-species hormones, that were more powerful and could be patented. Many clinical trials have shown that long-term combined oral HRT does have benefits, particularly the reduction of osteoporosis. However many of these studies have also shown that long-term oral combined HRT, does increase the incidence of breast cancer and blood clots. We know for sure that oral combined HRT should not be used as a preventive in women, who already have risk factors for cardiovascular disease, or who already have cardiovascular disease. The vast majority of these studies have used oral oestrogens that were cross-species oestrogens (equine), or too potent, and progesterone that was synthetic, and much more potent than our own natural progesterone. So it does not surprise me that the outcomes of these studies have been conflicting, often negative and disappointing, however one positive off-shoot is that we have learned how not to do it!

So now is the time for research to go back to the era of using natural hormones, to evaluate their long-term effects in quality-of-life issues, as well as the prevention of osteoporosis and cardiovascular disease. I feel very optimistic that further research into the use of natural hormones, will show far more positive outcomes for women than the use of synthetic hormones have shown. Of course this research takes 20 to 30 years to be completed, so we must start now.

It is now time to review outmoded, but commonly accepted treatment policies, for the menopause.

**New policies should take into account –**
- Current literature on all types of HRT, medical science and physiology
- A survey of doctors' experiences with HRT
- That every patient is unique, with important metabolic and hormonal characteristics
- The fact that we do not have long-term trials available for all types of HRT
- That the choice to take HRT belongs to the individual woman, and can only be made correctly by her with informed consent. No pressure should be exerted on a patient to take long term HRT for the prevention of chronic diseases.

**I think that updated and clear policies on HRT are needed for women in special subgroups, such as –**
- Women with breast cancer and uterine cancer

- Women who have risk factors (such as cardiovascular disease, liver disease, high blood pressure, obesity or diabetes, etc), but still want to take some form of HRT
- Women in the peri-menopause who suffer with estrogen dominance.

Doctors need more guidance from government health departments and academic institutions that do not have a vested financial interest in HRT. This guidance should be about the appropriate use of HRT, given the current climate of unreasonable litigation, which makes many doctors feel uncomfortable about prescribing HRT. This atmosphere of fear creates a barrier between doctors and patients, and can make doctors unduly conservative, which makes it harder for women to get help.

Since the outcome of the American WHI study was published in July 2002, many women have stopped taking their hormone replacement therapy; however many of them will return to their doctors, in subsequent years, complaining of symptoms of hormone deficiency, and wanting something done. Many women will think – 'Well, I do not feel safe taking hormones, but I can't live without them – help'!

**Doctors can rise to this challenge better, if they understand that –**

1. Every woman must be assessed as an individual, with unique hormonal and metabolic characteristics. These can be determined by a thorough history, medical examination and testing hormone levels accurately. The 'herd mentality' of stereotyping all menopausal women, so that every woman gets the same prescription, is no longer appropriate. This stereotyping of menopausal treatment, was reflected in the fact that in the year 2000, 46 million prescriptions were written for Premarin, making it the second most commonly prescribed drug in the USA.

Thankfully we will never see this mass-marketing of supermarket-brand name HRT again. What we will see is the use of tailormade, carefully designed, prescriptions of natural hormones for each woman. Not all women will need or want to take HRT, and they should not be pressurized to do so. However for those who want to, it is their right to be able to choose and receive the safest form of natural hormones.

2. Oral combined HRT, using synthetic or cross-species hormones, is no longer the gold standard that we compare all-types of hormone replacement therapy to. Lower doses of natural hormones, given by the safest route (such as transdermal hormones) will become the gold standard.

3. Women want to know about nutritional and complementary therapies. Doctors must keep an open mind if they want to keep patients under their umbrella of care. They must inform women of scams, such as homoeopathic hormones that purport to act as real hormones. These things are nothing more than money-wasters, and the alternative health industry must be just as accountable as drug companies.

4. It is the quality-of-life issues that are most important to women during the now relatively young years between the ages of 45 and 65. Women may need some form of natural HRT, on a short-term or intermittent basis, to provide a good quality-of-life during the years surrounding the menopause.

5. Today's woman is well educated and has high expectations she wants honesty and wants to be included in the decision-making process. This gives meaning to the term 'informed consent'.

In the mid-1980s the concept of the menopause as a disease was first introduced and promoted. This led to the commercially-motivated mass prescribing of inappropriate synthetic hormones, to prevent the diseases, not of the menopause, but of ageing. This has back-fired, and this type of HRT has been shown to have risks which outweigh its benefits. However, despite these negative outcomes, the use of all types of HRT is not doom and gloom.

We now stand at the beginning of a new era, where the menopause is no longer seen as a disease, but rather as a new, albeit sometimes challenging, phase of a woman's life. Natural hormones will be seen as a viable option to relieve the unpleasant, and sometimes debilitating, symptoms of the hormonal changes that occur in our bodies during the menopause. Natural hormone replacement therapy will be used appropriately, to enhance the quality of our mental, physical and sexual lives.

Wishing you good health and happiness

Sandra Cabot

Sandra Cabot MD

**Dr Sandra Cabot's Hormonal Advisory Service:**
provides assistance with diet, phytoestrogens and supplement
programmes to enhance your natural hormone prescription.
**www.weightcontroldoctor.com**
**www.whas.com.au**

*Contacts for pharmacies that compound Bio-identical Hormones;*
The International Academy of Compounding Pharmacists
email iacpinfo@iacprx.org or visit www.iacprx.org
Professional Compounding Centers of America
www.pccarx.com

**Books**
*Can't Lose Weight? Unlock The Secrets That Keep You Fat*
    Dr Sandra Cabot, SCB International Inc.
*Raw Juices Can Save Your Life*
    Dr Sandra Cabot, SCB International Inc.
*The Menopause Industry*
    Sandra Coney, 1994 Hunter House Publishing.

*What your doctor may not tell you about menopause*
  Dr John Lee, Warner Books.
*The Woman's Heart Book, The Complete Guide to Keeping Your*
  *Heart Healthy*
  New York, NY Penguin Books, Pashkow.
*Heal Cancer, Australia: Hill of Content*
  1993 Dr. Ruth Cilento.
*Always a Woman*
  New York, Bantam Books, 1982 Kaylan Pickford.
*Your Life In Your Hands – Understanding, Preventing and*
  *Overcoming Breast Cancer*
  Professor Jane Plant, Virgin Publishing

## HRT STUDIES

The WHI Study, The Risks and Benefits of Estrogen and Progestin in healthy post-menopausal women, *JAMA* 2002, July 17; 288:321–333

The PEPI Trial; The Postmenopausal Estrogen Progestin Interventions Trial, Effects of HRT on endometrial histology in postmenopausal women, *JAMA* 1996, February 7; 275(5):370–375

The PEPI Trial; The Postmenopausal Estrogen Progestin Interventions Trial, *JAMA* 1996, Nov. 6; 276(17):1430–32

The PEPI Trial; The Postmenopausal Estrogen Progestin Interventions Trial, *JAMA* 1997, May 21; 277(19):1515–17

A MacLennan, for the Australian Menopause Society 'Consensus Statement. Hormone Replacement Therapy and the Menopause', *Medical Journal of Australia* 155 (1991): 43–44

## MELATONIN

Wilson, S, et al, Melatonin augments the sensitivity of MCF–7 human breast cancer cells to tamoxifen in vitro, *Journal Clinical Endocrinology and Metabolism* 75;669–70, 1992

Pierpaoli, W, et al, Pineal control of aging; effect of melatonin and pineal grafting on aging mice, *Proc Nat Acad Sci* 91;787–791, 1994

Hardeland, R, et al, The significance of the metabolism of the neurohormone melatonin; antioxidant protection and formation of bioactive substances, *Neuro-Science and Behavioural reviews* 17;347–357, 1993

Hill, S, et al, Effect of the pineal hormone melatonin on the proliferation and morphological characteristics of human breast cancer cell (MCF7) in culture, *Can Res* 48;6121–26, 1988

Maestroni, G, et al, Role of the pineal gland in immunity. Circadian synthesis and release of melatonin, modulates the antibody response and antagonises the immunosuppressive effect of corticosterone, *J Neuroimmun* 3; 19–30, 1986

## PHYTOESTROGENS
### Soy

Adlercreutz H, Phytoestrogens: Epidemiology and a possible role in cancer protection, *Environmental Health Perspectives* 103, Suppl. 7:103–12, 1995

Ingram D, et al, Case-Control study of phytoestrogens and breast cancer, *The Lancet* 1997, Oct 4; 350:990–4

Kennedy A R, The evidence for soybean products as cancer preventive agents, *Journal of Nutrition* 125, 3 Suppl: 733S–43S, 1995

Albertazzi P, et al, The effect of dietary soy supplementation on hot flashes, *Obstetrics and Gynecology*, January 1988; Vol 91, No 1: 6–11

Messina M, The role of soy foods in preventing and treating chronic disease

Beckham N, Natural therapies for menopause and osteoporosis – a practitioner guide, 1997

Isoflavones in the Management of the Menopause; Proceedings from an Educational Meeting. *The Journal of the British Menopause Society*, Volume 7, Supplement 1, 2001

Adlercreutz H, et al, Phytoestrogens and Western diseases, *Ann Med* 1997; 29:95–120

Adlercreutz H, et al, Dietary phytoestrogens and the menopause in Japan, *The Lancet* 1992; 339:1233

Baber RJ, et al, A randomized placebo controlled trial of an isoflavone supplement and menopausal symptoms in women, *Climacteric* 1999; 2:85–92

Nachtigall LB, et al, The effect of isoflavones derived from red clover on vasomotor symptoms and endometrial thickness. Proceedings 81st Annual Meeting US Endocrine Society 1999; June 1999, San Diego

Arora A, et al, Antioxidant activities of isoflavones and their biological metabolites, *Arch Biochem Biophys* 1998; 356:133–41

Reinli K, Phytoestrogen content of foods – a compendium of literature values, *Nutrition and Cancer* 1996; 26(2):124–148

H Adlercreutz, T Fotsis et al, Determination of Urinary Lignans and Phytoestrogen Metabolites, *Journal of Steroid Biochemistry* 25, 5B, November 1986: 791–797

## PROGESTERONE

The PEPI Trial; The Postmenopausal Estrogen Progestin Interventions Trial, Effects of HRT on endometrial histology in postmenopausal women, *JAMA* 1996, February 7; 275(5):370–375

Affinito et al, *Maturitas Journal of the Climacteric and Postmenopause* 20 (1995); 191–198

Yu S, et al, Apoptosis induced by progesterone in human ovarian cancer cell line SNU-840, *J Cell Biochem* 2001; 82:445–451

Formby B, Wiley TS, Progesterone inhibits growth and induces apoptosis in breast cancer cells: Inverse effects on Bcl-2 and p53, *Ann Clin Lab Sci* 1998; 28:360–369

Shyamala G, Progesterone action in human breast cancer. 1995; *International Journal of Pharmaceutical Compounding.* www.iacprx.org/

Prior JC, Progesterone as a bone-trophic hormone, *Endocr Rev* 1990; 11:386–398

Baulieu EE, Schumacher M. Neurosteroids, with special reference to the effect of progesterone on myelination in peripheral nerves, *Multiple Sclerosis* 1997;3:105–112

Nilsen J, Brinton RD, Impact of progestins on estrogen induced neuro-protection: Synergy by progesterone and antagonism by medroxyprogesterone acetate, *Endocrinology* 2002; 143:205–212

## CARDIOVASCULAR DISEASE

Gordon T, et al, Menopause and coronary artery disease: The Framingham Study, *Ann Intern Med* 1978; 89:157–61

Heart and Stroke Facts 1996 Report, Canberra; National Heart Foundation of Australia, 1996

Heart and Stroke Facts 1995, Statistical Supplement, Dallas TX, American Heart Association, 1994

MJ Stampfer, GA Colditz, et al., Postmenopausal Estrogen Therapy and Cardiovascular Disease, *The New England Journal of Medicine* 325 (11) (12 September 1991): 756–762

R Bergstrom, M Falkeborn, I Persson, et al., 'Hormone Replacement Therapy and the Risk of Stroke: Follow-up of a Population-based Cohort in Sweden', *Archives of Internal Medicine* 153 (10) (24 May 1993): 1201–1209

R Buist, The Role of Nutrients in the Prevention of Heart Disease, Report to the seminar 'Nutrition in Disease Prevention', Sydney, Australia, Australian Council for Responsible Nutrition, 9 March 1992

## ESTROGEN

Tang M-X et al, Effect of estrogen during menopause on risk and age at onset of Alzheimer's disease, *The Lancet* 1996; 348:429–32

Vooijs GP et al, Review of the endometrial safety during intravaginal treatment with estriol, *Eur J Obstet Gynecol Reprod Biol* 1995; 62:101–106

J Studd et al., Estradiol and Testosterone Implants, *British Journal of Obstetrics and Gynaecology* 84 (1977): 314–315

Estrogen Level Score Chart, Prof. Chris Nordin, Institute of Medical and Veterinary Science, University of Adelaide, S.A.

**BREAST CANCER**

Cavalieri EI et al, Molecular origin of cancer: catechol estrogen-3, 4-quinones as endogenous tumor initiators, *Proc. Natl. Acad. Sci.* 1997;94:10937–42

Schairer C et al, Menopausal estrogen and estrogen-progestin replacement therapy and breast cancer risk, *JAMA* 2000; 283: 485–497

KK Steinberg et al, A meta-analysis of the effect of estrogen replacement therapy on the risk of breast cancer, *Journal of the American Medical Association* 265 (1991): 1985–1990

**OSTEOPOROSIS**

FS Kaplan, Osteoporosis: Pathophysiology and Prevention, in Clinical Symposia, Vol.39 (1) Ciba-Geigy Corporation, 1987, 1–32

MW Tilyard et al., Treatment of Postmenopausal Osteoporosis with Calcitriol or Calcium, *The New England Journal of Medicine* 326 (1992): 357–362

JC Stevenson et al., Effects of transdermal versus oral HRT on Bone Density in the spine and femur in postmenopausal women, *The Lancet* 336 No.II (1990): 265–269

# Glossary

**Adrenal glands** Two small glands situated on top of the kidneys that secrete various hormones, including epinephrine (adrenaline), cortisone and DHEA

**Anabolic steroids** Synthetic hormones that stimulate the growth of bone and muscle and have masculinizing effects on the body.

**Androgen** Sex hormones that promote the development of masculine characteristics, such as facial and body hair

**Antioxidant** A substance that protects cellular structures against oxidative damage. Well-known antioxidants include vitamins A, C, and E; beta-carotene; the minerals zinc and selenium; and the enzyme Superoxide Dismutase (SOD)

**Atrophy** Wasting or thinning of tissues or organs

**Autoimmune disease** A group of diseases produced by a malfunction of the immune system that causes the immune system to attack and inflame the body's own tissues and organs

**Cancer** A type of disease characterized by the rapid multiplication of abnormal cells, resulting in a malignant growth, or tumour, that may spread to, and invade, distant body parts

**Cancer chemotherapy** The administration of toxic chemical drugs into the body for the purpose of killing cancer cells

**Cardiovascular disease** Any disease of the circulatory system, which comprises the heart and blood vessels

**Cholesterol** A sterol that is a constituent of all animal cells. High levels of the bad LDL-cholesterol increase the risk of cardiovascular disease. Dietary cholesterol is found in fats and oils of animal origin. Cholesterol is made by the liver

**Circulation** The recurrent and continual movement of the blood through the heart and various blood vessels of the body

**Collagen** A fibrous protein that gives elasticity and strength to the skin, bones, cartilage, and connective tissues

**Curettage** The procedure of surgically scraping a body cavity (such as the uterus) to remove tissue, blood, or abnormal growths

**Deficiency** Lack or insufficiency of an essential substance

**Dowager's hump** A curve on the upper spine, below the neck, that forms as a result of compression fractures of the spinal vertebrae

**Endocrine system** The network of ductless glands that manufacture and secrete hormones into the bloodstream; these hormones affect the function of distant organs and tissues

**Endocrinology** The study and treatment of disorders of the glands and the hormones they secrete

**Endometrial ablation** A surgical procedure in which the inner lining of the uterus is destroyed by means of radio waves or a laser beam

**Endometriosis** A disorder in which the endometrial cells, which are normally confined inside the uterine cavity, become scattered around the outside the uterus, in the abdomen, and/or in the pelvic cavity. It usually results in pain, possibly severe pain, during menstruation

**Endometrium** The mucous membrane forming the inner layer, or lining, of the uterus

**Enzyme** Any of the proteins that catalyse or facilitate chemical reactions in cells. They are necessary to break down, or metabolize, nutrients, drugs and hormones

**Epidemiologist** A specialist who deals with the spread of diseases among populations

**Essential fatty acids** Fatty acids necessary for cellular metabolism; they cannot be produced by the body and must be supplied in the diet. Suitable sources are flaxseed oil, evening primrose oil, fish oil, and various seeds and nuts

**Fibroids** Non-cancerous growths in the uterus that consist of muscle and fibrous tissue

**Follicle Stimulating Hormone (FSH)** A hormone secreted by the pituitary gland that acts on the ovary, causing it to develop ripened follicles (eggs). These follicles produce oestrogen

**Genetic engineering** Man-made alteration in the genetic structure of cells, usually done for breeding purposes or to eradicate diseases, or to enable cells to synthesize chemicals or hormones

**Gland** *See* Endocrine system

**Heredity** The quality of being passed through the genes from the parents to their offspring, as characteristics or diseases

**Hormone** Any of the chemicals that are produced by various glands in the body, which are transported in the blood to affect distant cells and organs

**Hormone Replacement Therapy (HRT)** The administration of hormonal preparations (natural or synthetic), to make up for the decline of natural hormone production by various glands

**Hypertension** High blood pressure

**Hypothalamus** A major control centre of the brain that regulates temperature, appetite, thirst and the function of hormonal glands. It is situated at the base of the brain and is directly connected to the pituitary gland

**Hysterectomy** Surgical removal of the uterus

**Implant** A chemical substance or object that is surgically implanted into a part of the body

**Incontinence** The inability to restrain or control the discharge of urine or faeces

**Inflammation** A condition characterized by swelling, redness, heat and pain in any tissue. Inflammation may occur as a result of trauma, irritation, infection or imbalances in immune function

**Insomnia** The inability to sleep

**Libido** Sexual desire

**Menopause** The final cessation of menstruation; the last menstrual period. It is caused by failure of the ovaries

**Menstruation** The cyclic (usually monthly) discharge of blood from the non-pregnant uterus; also called the menstrual period

**Metabolism** The complex of chemical processes utilizing the raw materials of nutrients, oxygen and vitamins, along with enzymes, to produce energy for body functions

**Minerals** A group of inorganic substances which are essential for normal cellular metabolism, the structural integrity of bone, and the maintenance of life

**Mucous membrane** A lubricating membrane lining the internal surface of an organ such as the intestines, vagina or bladder, etc

**Naturopathic medicine** An approach to health care that utilizes the prevention and treatment of illnesses with naturally-occurring substances such as juices, vitamins, minerals and herbs

**Oestradiol** A natural oestrogen produced by the ovary. It is the most potent of all the three natural oestrogens

**Oestriol** A natural oestrogen made by the ovary. All the body's oestrogens eventually become broken down into oestriol, which is excreted from the body in the urine. Oestriol is the weakest of all the body's oestrogens

**Oestrogen** This is the collective term used for the three oestrogens produced by the ovary. Oestrogenic hormones are responsible for female characteristics such as the development of breasts and feminine curves, as well as menstruation

**Oestrogen Receptors** Physical structures on the cell membranes, which attract oestrogen, and respond to its effects

**Oestrone** A natural oestrogen produced in the ovary and the fat tissues, especially the fat in the lower segment of the body

**Osteoporosis** A very common disorder characterized by loss of bone mass, due to loss of minerals and collagen from the bone; it results in a porous condition of the bones and skeletal atrophy

**Ovaries** The female sex glands (gonads) located on each side of the uterus that produce eggs and sex hormones, including oestrogen and progesterone, as well as a smaller amount of androgens

**Palpitations** Irregular or excessively rapid heart beats

**Pap smear** A test in which cells are gently scraped from the cervix and smeared onto a glass slide for examination under a microscope. It is a screening test for cancer of the cervix

**Peak bone mass.** The ultimate or maximum amount of bone in the skeleton, usually achieved around the age of 30

**Pelvic floor muscles** The muscles that form the anatomical 'floor' of the pelvic cavity and give support to the pelvic organs, including the uterus, bladder and rectum

**Peri-menopausal** The years leading up to, during, and just after the menopause (roughly between the ages of 45 and 55)

**Pituitary gland** A mushroom-shaped gland that is connected by a stalk to the base of the brain. It manufactures many different hormones that in turn control other glands, such as the thyroid, the adrenal glands, the testicles and the ovaries

**Post-menopause** The period of time after the menopause

**Pre-menopause** The period of time leading up to the menopause. Generally four to five years long, it usually starts in the forties, but it can begin any time after the age of 35, and is characterized by hormonal imbalance

**Progesterone** A sex hormone secreted by the corpus luteum of the ovary that acts to prepare the uterus for the possibility of pregnancy. It has many health benefits in the female

**Progestogen** A synthetic form of the hormone progesterone, that is capable of producing menstrual bleeding

**Prolapse** The abnormal dropping or protrusion of a bodily organ or structure, most often the rectum (bowel), bladder, uterus or vagina

**Sex Hormone Binding Globulin (SHBG)** A protein in the blood that binds with and transports the sex hormones oestrogen, progesterone, and testosterone. When bound to SHBG, the sex hormones are inactive

**Stroke** A condition in which the blood supply to the brain is interrupted, causing malfunction of the brain. A stroke may be mild and transitory, with no lasting effects, or it may cause permanent brain damage resulting in a degree of disability or even death

**Testosterone** The primary sex hormone responsible for the development of masculine characteristics

**Thrombosis** The formation of a blood clot in a blood vessel

**Uterus** The female reproductive organ in which the fertilized egg implants, and develops into an embryo; also called the womb

**Vagina** The genital cavity from the uterus to the vulva

**Vertebrae** The bone segments that form the spinal column

**Vitamins** A group of food factors essential for cellular metabolism and the maintenance of life

**Vulva** The external female genitalia

Most of us are aware that fitness is important and that being fit is good for you. So, what is fitness? Basically, fitness is having the energy to perform your daily activities with enough energy left at the end of the day to enjoy your leisure time. To improve fitness for health and longevity we need to consider the following five areas:

- Cardiovascular fitness
- Muscular endurance
- Muscular strength
- Body fatness
- Flexibility

**Cardiovascular fitness** is the ability of the heart and lungs to supply the body with oxygen needed to convert food into energy. It also reduces the risk of coronary heart disease.

**Muscular endurance** is the ability of the muscles to work continuously with less fatigue. It also improves muscle tone.

**Muscular strength** helps protect the joints from injuries and allows daily activities to be performed without undue strain on the muscles.

**Body fatness** (composition) means a certain level of body fat is important, not only for appearance but also to help reduce the risk of heart disease, cancer and high blood pressure.

**Flexibility** helps prevent postural defects and back problems in later life due to lack of muscle elasticity. Regular stretching improves flexibility.

## Aerobic Exercise

Aerobic means 'with air'. That is, breathing in air and oxygen continually to supply oxygen to the working muscles. The activity needs to be continuous at an intensity that suits your fitness level. To ensure the exercise is, in fact, aerobic, remember the word FITT.

**Frequency**: at least three times a week; five times is better.
**Intensity**: exercise at 65–75 per cent of your maximum heart rate*.
**Time**: twenty minutes CONTINUOUS is the minimum, 30–60 minutes is better.
**Type**: type of exercise, aerobic classes, running, swimming, cycling, brisk walking, cross-country skiing, any activity that makes you huff and puff, and your heart beat strongly.
* Maximum heart rate is calculated by subtracting your age from 220.

With aerobic exercise the heart and lungs become stronger, which lessens the risk of heart disease. Fat particles may clog the inner walls of the arteries leading to the heart, with the possible result being a heart attack. In aerobic exercise the blood rushes through the arteries at speed, carrying away fatty particles for elimination.

**Aerobic exercise** is an excellent way to lose body fat. When exercise begins, the body uses its muscle glycogen (muscle food) stores first, keeping fat as a reserve fuel. After 20 minutes the muscle food has been used so the body has no choice but to draw on its stores of body fat for energy. Hence, the importance of doing continuous aerobic exercise for MORE than 20 minutes.

A good way to get aerobically fit is to attend aerobic classes. They keep you motivated while improving your strength and endurance.

## If You Don't Use It, You Lose It

Muscles need to be used! They need to be contracted to keep them strong, toned and healthy. When we use our muscles they become firm and shapely. When we don't use our muscles they become soft and flabby.

Let's take a look at toning and shaping. You may be familiar with abdominal exercises, push-ups, squats and knee bends. These are basic exercises that can use our own body weight to be effective. Another way of toning and shaping our body is through resistance training, whereby we contract our muscles against a variable resistance. That is, we can use free weights as in weight or resistance training. This kind of muscle shaping is very effective, and good results can be obtain in as short a period as six weeks, especially if the training is well programmed and monitored. Correct training can be done by people of any age—even if you're 90.

### The Benefits Of Muscle Training
1. Muscle training tones and strengthens muscles to improve appearance and make clothes look better.
2. Stronger muscles help protect joints against instability and injury.

3. If stretching is carried out before and after exercise, postural defects due to poor strength and flexibility are improved.
4. Muscle training improves muscular endurance, allowing muscles to work for daily activity.
5. Working through a full range of motion increases your flexibility, improves your mental functioning and also increases bone density, which in turn may prevent osteoporosis.
6. Muscles metabolize more internal energy when they are toned.

## Soft Exercises

Stiffness is a lack of suppleness or mobility, and gradual stiffness is part of the ageing process. This process can be slowed by regular stretching.

Stretching releases tension in the muscles, eliminating lactic acid and decreasing muscle tightness after exercise, bringing in nutrients and improving the blood supply to the muscles. It also assists in the co-ordination between muscle groups, improving posture.

Stretching is an effective way of refreshing a tired body and aids relaxation.

A fit healthy body has strength and stamina, suppleness and stability. Hard exercise develops strength and stamina, while softexercise develops suppleness and stability.

# Stretching

The aim of these stretching exercises is to improve flexibility and promote relaxation by stretching of the major muscle groups.

Remember to keep your breathing soft and rhythmic, and with every outward breath relax your body more and more. Over-stretching causes the muscles to shake, so relax the stretch and start again. If a position is painful to you, don't do that particular stretch. Each stretch should be held between 10 and 20 seconds. Take your time and enjoy!

**Follow the diagrams carefully.**

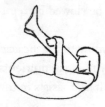

## Back Extensors
Curl into a ball.

## Quadriceps
Hold your left foot with your right hand and vice versa using the free hand to balance if necessary.

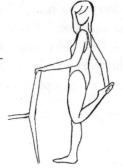

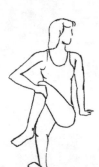

## Buttock Stretches
Keep both buttocks on the ground with your back straight.

Press against your knee as shown while turning your leg away from your body.

## Hamstrings

Keep your lower back pressed to the floor.

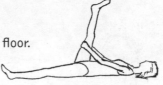

## Shoulder

Pull your elbow across to the opposite shoulder.

Hold your arm across your body with your thumb pointing towards the ground.

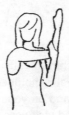
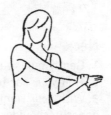

## Latissimus Dorsi

With one hand over the other, stretch forward as shown, hips in the air.

Lean your hips towards the side to be stretched.

Feel the stretch from shoulder blade to armpit.

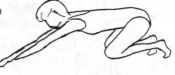

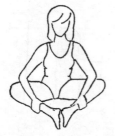

## Groin

Push your knees towards the floor. Don't bounce.

## Triceps

Place your behind your head and pull the elbow behind your head with the opposite hand.

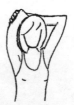

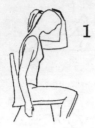 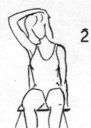 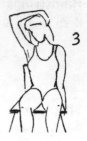

## Neck

1. Gently pull your chin to your chest.
2. Pull your ear to your shoulder.
3. With your right hand on your head, quarter turn it to the opposite shoulder and vice-versa.

Repeat the above.

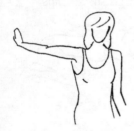

## Biceps

Hold on to a door at arm's length with your thumbs down.

Turn your body away from the arm and let your shoulder roll in.

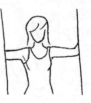

## Pectorals

Place your elbows against a doorway and lean your body forwards.

# Exercises

## Abdominal Curls

Lie on the floor with your knees bent.
Curl up and touch the top of your knees.
Keep your chin tucked into your neck.
Hips remain on the floor. Slowly return to floor.
Do not throw your head and shoulders up.

Pull with your abdominals.

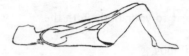 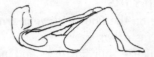

## Side Leg Raises

Lie on your side as shown, lifting your top leg to about 45° and
lowering it down again.

Flex your left foot, i. e. pull your toes towards your
shin, turn your foot with your big
toe towards the floor.

## Abdominal Obliques

Lie on the floor with your knees bent.

Place one hand on the floor next to your body and the other hand
behind your head.
Slightly raise your head off the
ground and move the elbow of the
hand behind your head towards your hip.

## Inner Leg Lifts

Lie on the floor as shown.

Bend slightly at the waist while
lifting your lower leg up and down.

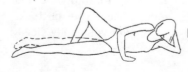

## Lower Abdominal Tucks

Keep your lower back pressed to the floor.
Lie on your back and place your arms on the floor next to your body with the palms down.

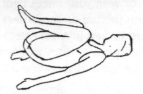

Bend your knees with your feet close to your buttocks.
Pull with your lower abdominals, rolling your knees to your chest and lifting your buttocks off the floor.

## Hip Lifts

Lie on the floor with your arms next to your body with the palms down.
Squeeze your buttocks and inner thighs.
Slightly lift your buttocks and the lower part of your back while clenching your buttocks.

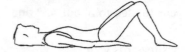

Rotate your pelvis upward. Do not lift your back, and rest on your shoulders.

## Triceps Extension

This can be done with your hands on the floor or on a step as shown, which will give a greater range of motion.

Rest your body weight on your arms, not legs.

Press up and down bending your elbows. Keep elbows slightly bent in the top position.

## Back Extension

Lie face down on the floor with your hands behind your head.
Lift your torso off the floor and squeeze your buttocks.
Lower your body slowly.

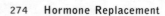

## Push Ups

Rest on your hands and knees with your feet in the air as shown.
Keep your body in a straight line throughout the movement with
your hands placed 10–15 cm wider than your shoulders.

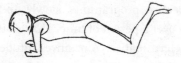

Keep your head up and lower
yourself to the floor.
Don't lie down and don't leave
your hips in the air.

Press up to the starting position but do not lock elbows.

## Calf Raises

Keep your knees and hips in a straight line.
Press right up on the ball of your foot.
Stretch your heels down as far as possible.
Return to the stretched position and
repeat. Don't bounce.

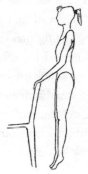

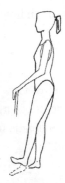

## Toe Taps

This exercise is simply pointing and flexing
your foot as shown.

## Side Arm Raises

Lift your arms from the side of your body parallel to the floor.
Keep your upper arm in line with your body, forearms slightly
forward, and bend your elbows.
Keep your elbows up and turn your thumbs
slightly to the floor.
Keeping your arms in this position,
lower them to your sides and repeat.
Added resistance (weights) may be used.

One of the most important factors to getting fit is consistency of effort. It is much better to do something every day rather than to kill yourself in one great effort, which can be detrimental and stressful to the body, putting you off exercise all together. (Inch by inch is a cinch.) Begin your exercise programmes slowly and steadily, increasing your intensity over a period of time. That time will depend on your efforts and determination. A positive attitude is not only necessary in every day activities, it's an essential ingredient of your exercise routine.

You can read many books on fitness, longevity or how to prolong the ageing process but it all comes down to one thing, you have to get off the chair and MOVE! It's up to you! No one will come and knock on your door and make you fit. No pill or potion will give you that feeling of fitness that you'll achieve through discipline, determination and effort. The control to have the body you want is within your power. You make the decision on how you look, how healthy you are and how vital you'll be.

So there's no time like the present! Begin now and get fit for a lifetime. Don't take a lifetime to get fit, because if you don't use it, you will lose it. The power to have a strong, healthy, vital, energetic body, with a positive, passionate outlook on life is up to you!

# Reference Values of Hormone Levels in Saliva Samples

These values were developed by Aeron Laboratories in the U. S. for their own testing of salivary hormone levels. Each laboratory develops their own reference ranges, and you should not intermix values from different laboratories.

**Ranges of Oestradiol levels in saliva** (for those with and without HRT supplementation) are outlined below.

Oestradiol is measured in pg/ml. Progesterone is measured in ng/ml

| OESTRADIOL | | PROGESTERONE | |
|---|---|---|---|
| **Not on HRT** | | | |
| *Premenopausal* | | *Premenopausal* | |
| follicular | 0.5–5 | follicular | <0.1 |
| midcycle | 3–8 | luteal | 0.1–0.5 |
| luteal | 0.5–5 | | |
| Postmenopausal | <1.5 | Postmenopausal | |
| **Supplemented with HRT** | | | |
| Oral Replacement* | 2–20 | Oral Replacement* | 0.1–0.5 |
| Hormone Patch* | 1–5 | Transdermal cream* | 1.0–10 |
| Transdermal Cream* | 10–50 | | |

• Ranges represent levels 8–12 hours after last dose or application of HRT

### Age and Sex Specific Ranges for DHEA in Saliva.

These are Unsupplemented A.M. Ranges. These units are in pg/ml

| FEMALE | | MALE | |
|---|---|---|---|
| Age | Range | Age | Range |
| 20–29 | 106–300 | 20–29 | 137–336 |
| 30–39 | 77–217 | 30–39 | 82–287 |
| 40–49 | 47–200 | 40–49 | 68–221 |
| 50–59 | 38–136 | 50–59 | 49–177 |
| 60–69 | 36–107 | 60–69 | 40–158 |
| 70–79 | 32–99 | 70–79 | 35–135 |
| >80 | 33–90 | >80 | 37–106 |

DHEA levels in saliva reflect active DHEA and not DHEA-S. Patients on transdermal DHEA creams may have high DHEA levels

### Age and Sex Specific Ranges for Testosterone in Saliva.

These are Unsupplemented A.M. Ranges. These units are in pg/ml

| FEMALE | | MALE | |
|---|---|---|---|
| Age | Range | Age | Range |
| 20–29 | 17–52 | 20–29 | 42–145 |
| 30–39 | 15–44 | 30–39 | 53–114 |
| 40–49 | 13–37 | 40–49 | 41–104 |
| 50–59 | 12–34 | 50–59 | 36–96 |
| 60–69 | 12–35 | 60–69 | 32–86 |
| 70–79 | 11–34 | 70–79 | 31–81 |
| | | >80 | 26–54 |

### Unsupplemented Female & Male Melatonin Ranges.

Units of measurement are in pg/ml.

| Time: | 10PM | 3AM | 7AM | 12 NOON |
|---|---|---|---|---|
| Mean: | 1 +/- 2 | 39 +/- 6 | 6 +/- 2 | 1 +/- 1 |
| Range: | 1–26 | 5–66 | 1–28 | 0.5–3 |

### Salivary Cortisol Ranges for Women and Men

| Cortisol levels in saliva reflect the active unbound hormone. Cortisol is measured in ng/ml | |
|:---:|:---:|
| A.M. | 1.0–8.0 |
| P.M. | 0.1–1.0 |

The term 'unsupplemented' means not on any form of Hormone Therapy or HRT.

## References

1) Ellison, P, Measurement of salivary progesterone, Ann NY *Acad Sci* 1992;161–176
2) Lipson, S and Ellison, P, Development of protocols for the application of salivary steroid analysis to field conditions, *American Journal of Human Biology*: 1989;1:249–255
3) Dabbs, JM, Salivary testosterone measurements: Collecting, storing and mailing saliva samples, *Physiology & Behaviour* 1990;49:815–817
4) Vinning RF, McGinley RA, The Measurement of Hormones in Saliva: Possibilities and Pitfalls, *J Steroid Biochem* 1987;27:81–94

# Make
# www.thorsonselement.com
# your online sanctuary

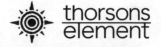